# Gut Feelings

## Disorders of Gut-Brain Interaction and the Patient-Doctor Relationship

# Gut Feelings

## Disorders of Gut-Brain Interaction and the Patient-Doctor Relationship

A GUIDE FOR PATIENTS AND DOCTORS

Douglas A. Drossman, MD

Johannah Ruddy, MEd

DROSSMANCARE

DrossmanCare Chapel Hill, NC 2021

In Collaboration with and Endorsed by the Rome Foundation

## DOUGLAS A. DROSSMAN, MD

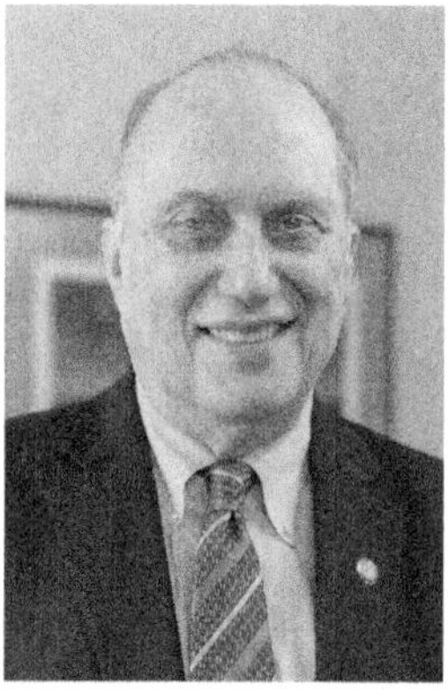

*Professor Emeritus of Medicine and Psychiatry*
*University of North Carolina at Chapel Hill*

*President Emeritus and Chief of Operations*
*of the Rome Foundation*

*President, Center for Education and Practice*
*of Biopsychosocial Care (DrossmanCare)*
*and Drossman Gastroenterology*

DR. DROSSMAN is trained in gastroenterology and psychiatry and was the founder and co-director of the Center for Functional GI and Motility Disorders at the University of North Carolina. He is an internationally recognized scientist, clinician, and educator in DGBI and communication skills training. He has written over 500 peer-reviewed scientific articles, published 15 books, and was awarded numerous federal research grants. He is the founder, former president, and current COO of the Rome Foundation. As president of DrossmanCare, he produces educational videos and develops workshops and training programs in communication skills. His internationally recognized gastroenterology practice receives patients with difficult to diagnose and manage DGBI.

## JOHANNAH RUDDY, MEd

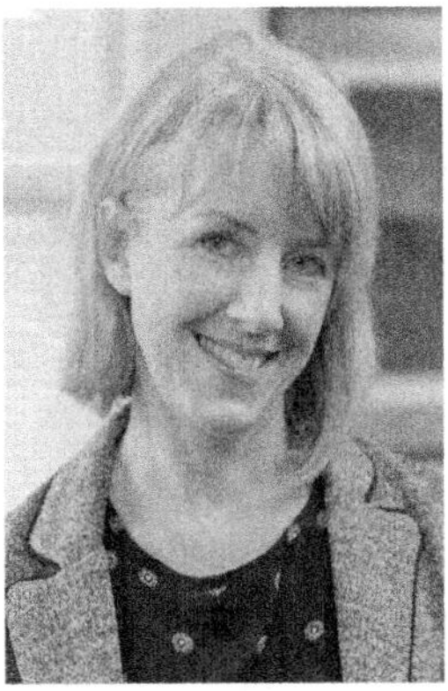

*Executive Director of the Rome Foundation*

*Secretary-Treasurer of the Center for Education and Practice of Biopsychosocial Care (DrossmanCare)*

MS. RUDDY is a patient and patient advocate with a background in education and a career in nonprofit management. As Executive Director of the Rome Foundation, she coordinates operations and educational programs. With DrossmanCare, Ms. Ruddy facilitates workshops in patient-centered care and is a simulated patient in videos on communication skills. Ms. Ruddy can articulate her experiences in a way that educates doctors and motivates patients to self-actuate and assume responsibility in their care. In this regard, her social media presence is well recognized, and she has published four peer-reviewed articles in scientific journals on patient advocacy and the importance of the patient perspective in medical education.

DROSSMANCARE



*Copy Editor:* Corinna Fales
*Illustrator and Graphic/Cover Designer:* Jerry Schoendorf
*Project Assistant:* Jennie Rambo
*Text Designer and Compositor:* Julie Allred, BW&A Books

*Front cover images:*
Photo 97023240 © Sebnem Ragiboglu | Dreamstime.com
Photo 43077523 © Gpointstudio | Dreamstime.com
Illustration 63208955 © Alexander Pokusay | Dreamstime.com
Photo 133422924 © Gballygiggs | Dreamstime.com
Photo 85187855 © Monkey Business Images | Dreamstime.com

ISBN 978-0-578-75966-1 (paperback with color images)
ISBN 978-0-578-75968-5 (paperback)
ISBN 978-0-578-75967-8 (ebook)
Library of Congress Control number: 2020921273

First Edition

*This book is dedicated to George Engel*
*who developed the concept of the Biopsychosocial Model,*
*to the many members of the Rome Foundation*
*whose mission is to "Improve the Lives of Patients*
*with Disorders of Gut-Brain Interaction,"*
*and to our spouses Debbie Drossman and Bryan Ruddy,*
*who supported us through the creation of this book.*

# Contents

# Foreword by Lin Chang, MD

Over 20 years ago when I was a junior faculty member at UCLA, I participated in a panel discussion at a conference symposium moderated by Dr. Doug Drossman on the importance of the patient-doctor relationship in managing patients with irritable bowel syndrome (IBS). It was my first introduction to Dr. Drossman's thoughtful and insightful approach of the optimal ways physicians can communicate with patients. I found myself having a lot of thoughts and comments on this topic. A day or two later, Dr. Drossman's physician assistant ran into me at the conference and suggested that I come visit them in North Carolina because I seem to be very interested in learning how to develop a therapeutic patient-doctor relationship. I took her up on this offer and I visited Dr. Drossman and saw patients with him. It was there that I really learned how to actively listen to them, ask thoughtful and relevant questions, understand and appreciate the patient's experience and perspective, recognize the importance of continuity of care and supportive reinforcement, and to be patient. Dr. Drossman taught me the biopsychosocial approach to Disorders of Gut-Brain Interaction (DGBI). The way he skillfully talked to patients, explained complex biological processes to patients so that they understood them, and negotiated a mutually agreeable management plan that empowered the patient was enlightening to me. He has been a mentor to me ever since then. We have written papers together on optimizing the patient-doctor relationship, conducted communication skills workshops, and work together in the Rome Foundation. I will be eternally grateful for the mentorship and training he has generously provided me so that I can more capably take care of patients. Subsequently, I have been able to train students, trainees, and other physicians how to communicate more skillfully with patients to improve health outcomes and satisfaction. I always tell people that Dr. Drossman taught me how to take care of patients.

Dr. Drossman and Johannah Ruddy have formed a synergistic partnership, educating both patients and healthcare providers about patient and doctor perspectives in DGBI and how to successfully build and nurture a therapeutic patient-doctor relationship. Johannah bravely recounts her medical history and the negative experiences she endured as a patient, but also how she learned about her IBS, how to manage her symptoms, and most importantly, find her voice and advocate for herself. Dr. Drossman deftly explains the ten ways doctors can enhance the patient-doctor relationship and provide patient-centered care. Together they provide scientific evidence that explains the etiology and symptoms of DGBI, and they also share what patients and doctors should know in order to maximize their partnership in patient care. Their book is a rich resource of information for patients, healthcare providers, and the general public. I have no doubt that you will feel enlightened reading this similar to how I felt when I visited Dr. Drossman so many years ago.

*Lin Chang, MD*
*Vice-Chief, Vatche and Tamar Manoukian Division of Digestive Diseases*
*Program Director, UCLA GI Fellowship Program*
*Co-Director, G. Oppenheimer Center for Neurobiology of Stress and Resilience*
*David Geffen School of Medicine at UCLA*
*Los Angeles, CA*

# Foreword by Jan Tack, MD, PhD

**THE PRACTICE OF MEDICINE** is rapidly transforming through the implementation of technical innovations and facilities. These have led to more accurate diagnoses and therapeutic innovations, but they also require new skills from physicians and have profoundly altered the doctor-patient relationship. Computer screens now occupy the space between the patient and doctor, apps monitor health parameters, and websites provide information on health, diseases, and treatments. Through these innovations and primarily because of the increasing time pressure on physicians and other healthcare providers, time devoted to the doctor-patient interaction has dramatically decreased. While healthcare spending increased more than 20-fold over the last decades, the average office visit time dropped by almost 75%. These numbers might raise the impression that direct interaction between patients and doctors is not so important after all. In a technology-driven view on medicine, the power is in numbers and images reporting test results, and anything beyond these aspects is redundant.

There is ample evidence of the opposite: effective communication between doctors and patients remains the cornerstone of disease management. While technology and the vast medical knowledge basis determine the accuracy of the diagnosis and the evidence base for the treatment plan, the communication secures the trust and engagement of the patient in the process, both short and long term. It also provides a basis for acceptance of side effects or less satisfactory outcomes. For the doctor, there are also benefits related to good communication with patients, including enhanced job satisfaction and prevention from burnout.

The role of effective patient-doctor communication is of even higher importance in disorders lacking diagnostic tests to make the diagnosis, such as the disorders of gut-brain interaction, previously referred to as functional gastrointestinal disorders. We define these conditions by a constellation of symptoms, the Rome Criteria, in the absence of a measurable diagnostic marker. Recognition of the symptom pattern to establish a diagnosis depends entirely on good history taking, which depends on a good patient-doctor relationship. Furthermore, it is well documented that after communicating the diagnosis, the quality of the patient-doctor interaction is a determinant of positive long-term outcomes.

In this book, two eminent experts, on either end of the patient-physician relationship, build on their personal experience and knowledge to express their views on patient-centered care. The framework for their description of the pivotal role of good patient-doctor communication is that of the disorders of gut-brain interaction. Johannah Ruddy, who wrote the patient perspective aspects in this book, is the Executive Director of the Rome Foundation, an independent nonprofit organization whose mission is to improve the lives of people with disorders of gut-brain interaction. This function, with the explicit focus on patient benefit, already puts her in an authoritative and privileged position to reflect the patient perspective. As is clear from her candid testimony in the book, she has also personally experienced the harmful effects of a callous patient-doctor interaction in a setting of debilitating chronic abdominal symptoms. Her extensive negative experience in interacting with the medical field took a dramatically favorable turn after consulting with Dr. Douglas Drossman. From that role, she experienced a lack of stigmatization, learned that the symptoms were taken seriously, and engaged in a quality patient-doctor interaction. These fundamental elements led her to gain control of the symptoms that had dominated her life for a decade.

Dr. Douglas Drossman, who wrote the physician sections of this book, is the founder of the Rome Foundation. He was instrumental in enabling the current recognition of disorders of gut-brain interaction as relevant clinical entities instead of older views of these entities as "imagined" or "not worth treating." Under his guidance, the Rome Foundation published diagnostic criteria and contributed considerably to the current concepts of these disorders, and how they can be diagnosed and managed in clinical practice. He also contributed descriptions of the major disorders of gut-brain interaction and how they are diagnosed and treated in the book. The Rome Foundation not only advocates state-of-the-art classical pharmacological therapies targeting the gastrointestinal tract. It also advocates the appropriate use of neuromodulators and behavioral or psychological treatments for these conditions.

While the book is written focusing on disorders of gut-brain interaction, its content has relevance to medicine in the broad sense. The importance of quality communications in medicine is not restricted to the gastroenterology field. Hence, the sections on how to use communication skills to optimize the patient-doctor relationship (and expandable to the patient-healthcare provider relationship) are of interest to anyone active in a healthcare setting. The recommendations and learning points address not only verbal communication but also the nonverbal aspects of the patient-doctor interaction. The recommendation section ends with 14 action points for daily practice. The book also gives guidance to patients on how to express themselves and what they can do to get the most out of patient-healthcare provider encounters.

My hope for the future is that the non-technical aspects of the patient-doctor encounter gain recognition for its merits and value. The book *Gut Feelings: Disorders of Gut-Brain Interaction and the Patient-Doctor Relationship: A Guide for Patients and Doctors* is an indispensable companion for providers as well as patients, who want to improve the quality and outcomes of health care. I applaud the authors for an outstanding and impressive book, and hope you will find an enjoyable and enriching reading experience.

*Jan Tack, MD, PhD*
*President, Rome Foundation*
*Head of Gastroenterology and Hepatology Division,*
*Leuven University Hospitals*
*Professor of Medicine, Leuven University*

# Preface by Douglas A. Drossman, MD

**WHAT A GREAT PLEASURE** to write this book; it is the culmination of decades of learning, teaching, and patient care. As I look back, it is hard to see how these seemingly disparate life experiences, neither anticipated nor fully understood by me at the time, came together in the way they did.

I always wanted to be a doctor. Perhaps it was a product of my culture and the subtle influence of my parents. I never knew that my father wanted to be a doctor, but because he had to support his family during the Depression, he never had the opportunity. I suspect he unconsciously influenced my career choice.

After medical residency during the Vietnam era, I went into the Air Force as an internist and saw many patients for brief visits. I began to realize that the medical symptoms patients conveyed to me often seemed unrelated to x-rays and laboratory findings. In the real world, I learned that much of my medical training just didn't fit. I also started "moonlighting"—working off-hours at a Women's Health Clinic, where I developed an understanding of the anorectal and pelvic floor structures and their dysfunction. That clinical experience influenced my knowledge of rectal and pelvic pain syndromes and constipation, which I brought to my future work in gastroenterology.

During my time in the Air Force, I heard about George Engel in Rochester, NY, who soon became my mentor. He coined the term Biopsychosocial Model, which became the driving force of my career. Dr. Engel was an internist and psychoanalyst who set up a training program to teach what was then called psychosomatic medicine. My growing concern about the disconnect between symptoms and medical findings drew me to his program. Also, he was considered a master medical interviewer. I recall him diagnosing what was later confirmed to be a thalamic tumor of the brain based on the quality of the pain the patient reported; I guess he preceded by decades the TV doctor "House." My learning with him allowed me to develop and expand my interview skills to improve my ability to acquire even subtle medical and biopsychosocial data. It also helped me to understand the patient's inner world and illness experience entirely differently. I now realized why objective medical tests were not sufficient to explain the patient's symptoms.

When I started my GI fellowship in 1976 at the University of North Carolina, I employed this new knowledge with my patients, and I believe this led to a different experience than my peers had. I remember interviewing patients before I was to endoscope them and predicted, with reasonable success, which ones would have an ulcer and which ones would have negative findings. Like my peers, I enjoyed learning about "organic" diseases like peptic ulcers, which were very common (before *H. pylori* and acid-blocking drugs), and inflammatory bowel disease. However, I was drawn to the functional GI disorders, an area that no one seemed to understand or care about. These disorders became the focal point for my developing interest in the connection between brain and gut.

In my early academic career at UNC, I met my second mentor, Don Powell, the GI division chief. While he didn't fully understand my evolving interests in functional GI disorders, he taught me how to write articles and to teach. A pivotal moment occurred when the journal *Gastroenterology* was starting a new teaching series, and its editor asked Don to write a review article. Don asked me to co-author, and I chose the topic of irritable bowel syndrome (IBS). That publication in 1977 was the first biopsychosocial article in the gastroenterology field. It incorporated the clinical features, motility, and psychosocial aspects of IBS into one review. The article was widely circulated and well received, and it propelled me into making the functional GI disorders my career choice.

Don also taught me to apply my ideas to research. Many investigators received training in epidemiology or basic sciences and then sought to find ways to apply this knowledge in research. Don taught me to do things differently. First, I was to reach down and explore what I learned from my patients. From this information, I would develop my research questions, then the tools to answer them would follow. By taking that approach, I was able to acquire NIH funding on novel research areas. I tried to reconcile why some people said IBS patients were "crazy," and others believed these patients had "real" symptoms. I was fortunate to receive an NIH grant on my first try to study IBS patients who went to doctors, those with IBS who had never been to doctors, and healthy subjects. It was a perfect model to learn the influence of stress and psychosocial factors on illness. The studies showed that these factors weren't part of IBS *per se*, but they worsened the symptoms and led them to seek health care. So the concept of individuals with IBS being "crazy" was debunked; instead, stress factors influenced symptom severity, patient behavior, and the decision to see doctors. My interviewing skills helped me to learn that many women with chronic GI symptoms had a history of early abuse and trauma, but they did not tell their doctors. The findings from my next NIH grant showed that up to half of the women who came to the GI clinic had a history of abuse. Furthermore, the abuse had severe adverse effects on GI health and clinical outcomes. The relationship between abuse and GI pain was later confirmed when we did brain imaging research. We also learned that abuse history didn't cause these disorders as some had thought, but it influenced how patients experienced and coped with the illness. Now it was becoming important to find the treatments. I was fortunate to receive the first NIH grant to study the benefit of cognitive-behavioral therapy and desipramine (a neuromodulator) for irritable bowel syndrome. Doing this type of research was difficult because there were no questionnaires at the time to measure the impact of the illness on symptom severity or quality of life. So my research group developed and validated many of the questionnaires that are even used to this day.

My growing disillusion with the scientific understanding of these disorders, the failure of traditional approaches to grasp their negative impact on patient health, and the dissatisfaction of doctors treating these patients encouraged me to seek out colleagues to try to impact and resolve these issues. In the late 1980s, a group of like-minded clinicians and scientists, including William Whitehead, W. Grant Thompson, Enrico Corazziari, and Nicholas Talley, formed the Functional Brain-Gut Research Group of the American Gastroenterological Association. We promoted educational programs in functional GI disorders and supported research in the field. Shortly after that, in 1990, the group coalesced to form the Rome Foundation to develop diagnostic criteria and guidelines to study these patients further. We contributed to advancing the field of functional GI disorders and most recently changed the name to Disorders of Gut-Brain Interaction, which legitimized them for patients and clinicians. I need to thank my wife, Debbie, who supported my efforts in this work and was instrumental in influencing me to write the first Rome book.

Along with this research was my clinical interest in understanding and communicating better with patients. In the mid-1990s, my friend and colleague Mack Lipkin formed an organization, the American Academy of Physician and Patient (AAPP), now called the Academy of Communication in Health Care, which I joined as a faculty facilitator. The group ethic incorporated many of George Engel's teaching about interviewing and the relationship skills delineated by Carl Rogers. Dr. Rogers' person-centered approach influenced psychotherapy (client-centered therapy), teaching (student-centered learning), and clinical practice (patient-centered care). In this program I learned how to apply Mack's facilitation skills in working with groups, and that guided me in my future training programs. I also became close friends with Dennis Novack, learning from him and other faculty such as Tony Suchman and Penny Williamson; all of them went on to distinguish themselves in this emerging area of healthcare education. The total experience was eye-opening, and I continued throughout my career to teaching these techniques to clinicians and faculty at medical programs.

I brought this work into gastroenterology and gave lectures and held workshops on communication skills. I also formed the Center for Education and Practice of Biopsychosocial Care (DrossmanCare). To reach a larger audience, DrossmanCare produced teaching videos currently used by the Rome Foundation and many other groups.

The final element that brought together my work was collaborating with Johannah Ruddy, the co-author of this book. Johannah came to the Rome Foundation in 2017 as the Executive Director. Also, Johannah is a patient and patient advocate, as discussed in this book. Our professional association profoundly enhanced my educational approach to training doctors in communication skills by actively bringing in the patient's perspective. Johannah can articulate her experiences in a way that educates doctors and motivates patients to self-actuate and assume responsibility in their care. She also helped me to understand patient perspectives to a degree I had not previously considered. Finally, our collaboration has allowed us to work together to offer patient education in a way that reaches them at their experience level. This partnership wholly enriches this book.

What we have created is a learning experience for patients and doctors. Several key elements make this book unique:

- A conceptual understanding of the history, philosophy, and scientific basis for the biopsychosocial model, the brain-gut axis, and Disorders of Gut-Brain Interaction (DGBI)
- A comprehensive review of all the DGBI, including their definition, pathophysiology (how the disorder occurs), diagnosis, and treatment, based on the guidance of the Rome Foundation
- A learning program to improve communication skills and optimize the patient-doctor relationship
- Guidelines for the doctor on how to approach the diagnosis and treatment of DGBI
- A listing of top-tier clinical programs in the USA and internationally that treat patients with DGBI
- Enhancements to the learning experience:
    - Availability in hard copy and online formats
    - Links to videos that supplement and add to the information in the book
    - A comprehensive glossary
    - An appendix that lists the Rome IV diagnostic criteria for all the DGBI
    - An up-to-date bibliography of peer-reviewed publications.

I hope you will find this book informative and meaningful.

*Douglas A. Drossman, MD*

# Preface by Johannah Ruddy, MEd

When I was a little girl, I was the one who was quick to be the "helper" in any situation. My earliest memories are of working in the kitchen with my mother and grandmother, baking and cooking for the family or helping with laundry, cleaning, and other household chores. In high school, I was voted "Most Humanitarian Student," and in college, I volunteered and served in many capacities throughout the community. So, it was not a surprise to anyone that I fell in love with nonprofit work and education, both finding a home in my heart and allowing me the chance to excel at giving to others and creating a positive impact on the world. As I grew in my career, nonprofit management, and education, I found new ways to give back and provide help to those I served.

With every job, I have found opportunities to go above and beyond in my role. I love the opportunity to find the needs and then meet them. This has become woven into who I am as a human, woman, wife, and mother and is a core value in my life.

My background sets the stage for where I find myself now. As the Executive Director of the Rome Foundation and a GI patient advocate, I am in a unique position to reach a new audience in a different way. As a GI patient myself, I can uniquely relate to the myriad of emotions and situations that many patients encounter in their health journey. Because of this perspective, I have found a platform that is unlike others that I have had. While I have been impactful in the past working with patients living with heart disease, cancer, and muscular dystrophy or families facing homelessness, incarceration, or drug addiction, I have never experienced those issues personally. My attempts to help came from the outside looking in and hoping that my work would have an impact.

This time it is different. It is personal, raw, rough, and real. Everything that you will read in this book, I have experienced; now I can speak to you, patient to patient or patient to doctor, in a meaningful way.

Over the past decade of my health journey, I have learned a lot about how the health system views patients with chronic illness. I see their role in perpetuating the very real stigma that is attached to DGBI, such as IBS, and the impact of these conditions on one's quality of life. Since working with the Rome Foundation and DrossmanCare, I have been able to understand better the role that the dualistic model of patient care has had in the mismanagement of these patients. I can see how patients can play an active role in their medical care and find the symptom management strategies that they need to regain control and live a better life.

I hear from patients every day via email or through social media. They relay their stories of chronic illness, their frustration at the system that has left them broke, hopeless, and with no answers. I hear from physicians who are frustrated with a system that doesn't allow them to care for their patients in a meaningful way. The demands for them to spend more time on administrative tasks, instead of direct patient care, lead them to become fatigued and many burn out. It is a great honor to be a sounding board for patients and clinicians alike, to be a resource, and to offer hope and support.

All this leads to the evidence that the current model of healthcare delivery is broken and not benefitting patients or clinicians. The likelihood may be that this will not change for the better in my lifetime. So what can we do in this current situation to improve outcomes? You'll read more about what Dr. Drossman and I recommend from both of our unique perspectives, so I don't want to spoil the ending for you! I will leave you with one nugget of advice here. Patients and clinicians who engage with these disorders from a biopsychosocial perspective can work to improve their communication skills and engage collaboratively on the care that will improve the clinical outcome.

This takes me to my co-author, Dr. Douglas Drossman. If you have ever had the pleasure of meeting Dr. Drossman, you would probably describe him as a somewhat quiet, sarcastic, and soft-spoken guy who is quick to share his thoughts on the latest British drama series he is watching or a humorous, poop-themed pun. Working so closely with him, I find him to be these things, as well as a kind and well-meaning mentor and friend. When I first met Dr. Drossman in 2017, I was overwhelmed by his immense knowledge of the field, his impressive CV of research and publications, and his impressive legacy of establishing both the Rome Foundation and DrossmanCare. I found myself learning immediately from him about all things DGBI and the importance of communication skills to the practice of medicine. With my background in health-based nonprofits and education, I was impressed at what he has spent his life creating as a gift to the field and patients alike.

It was in 2019 that we began discussing the need for a patient book on DGBI, communication skills, self-advocacy, and the distinct but equally important roles of the patient and the physician. I also heard from patients of their great desire to have scientifically relevant and evidence-based education available that they could understand and access easily. We decided to write a book that would meet this need, but we would uniquely write it for patients and physicians alike. However, with our busy schedules, we did not know when we might get to it. Little did we know that 2020 would be the year that the universe provided the time, because of the global pandemic. All the international meetings that would have filled our calendars in a typical year were canceled. Suddenly we found ourselves with a block of time to devote to this book.

This book was not easy to write for either of us. It is the combination of much time, effort, energy, and emotion. We wanted it to be impactful for anyone who reads it to provide education, support, and encouragement that we all need when we live with a chronic illness. I am forever grateful to Dr. Drossman for pushing me to do this book with him and also to dig deep and share the personal and emotional aspects of my life and my illness journey to help others. Being vulnerable and sharing painful parts of one's life is not an easy process. I found a sense of healing through the process, though, and I hope that my story will resonate with you and let you know that you are not alone.

Looking back on my life and my professional career, I find that I have come full circle. I now can tap into my life experience and proudly advocate for patients with gastrointestinal disorders with a thorough understanding of their experience. I can educate patients and clinicians about these disorders, and provide a safe place for support and hope for all who need it. I am proud of this book and what Dr. Drossman and I continue to create to impact the lives of patients and clinicians positively, and I look forward to new and exciting endeavors in the future.

Finally, I have to thank a few people in my life who have provided the support and love that has carried me to this point. To my husband Bryan and my two sons, Tyler and Connor, you are my life and my love, and I would be lost without you.

I hope that you enjoy this book, and I look forward to hearing from you personally in the future.

*Johannah Ruddy, MEd*

# Acknowledgments

**THE AUTHORS ARE MOST GRATEFUL** to Corinna Fales for her insights and editing skills to bring us to this finished product. It was a delight to work with her. We also would like to thank Jennie Rambo for technical and administrative assistance, Jerry Schoendorf for support with the graphic arts, and Julie Allred for her help in the composition of this book. Importantly, we want to thank the Rome Foundation Board of Directors and members for their commitment to teaching doctors and promoting the clinical care of patients with DGBI. We also would like to thank the Rome Foundation Research Institute for supporting high-quality research to advance the field of DGBI.

# GUT FEELINGS

Disorders of Gut-Brain Interaction
and the
Patient-Doctor Relationship

# Introduction

*"Man should strive to have his intestines relaxed all the days of his life."*
—Moses Maimonides (Rambam), 1134–1204 AD

*"A good set of bowels is worth more to a man than any quantity of brains."*
—Josh Billings (Henry Wheeler Shaw), 1818–1885 AD

Nowadays, doctors can only spend about a fifth of the time for their office visits as compared to what they spent decades ago. Furthermore, to make diagnoses, now they often rely on tests, rather than on face-to-face dialog and physical examinations.[1] While medical tests are a terrific tool for revealing organic (structural) abnormalities in the body that identify disease, most patients complain about ***illness***, which involves symptoms that are not necessarily determined by testing. Illness refers to the personal experience of ill health or bodily dysfunction, which may relate to current or previous disease in conjunction with psychosocial, family, and cultural influences. ***Disease***, on the other hand, refers to abnormalities in the structure and function of organs and tissues that are externally verifiable by tests like blood work, x-rays, endoscopy, or a CT scan. The difference between illness and disease is the basis for the difficulties we have had in forming a correct medical understanding of Disorders of Gut-Brain Interaction (DGBI). It also contributes to the dilemma we face in a dualistic healthcare system that erodes the patient-doctor relationship and negatively impacts patient care.

Western medicine is influenced by a concept called dualism, which conceives of the mind and body as separate. The result of this thinking is that "organic," or structurally based diseases, are considered real and authentic, and patients who have them are deemed to have "rightful" suffering. In contrast, patients who suffer from functional (non-structural) illnesses such as DGBI, chronic pain, fibromyalgia, and chronic fatigue (which are defined by symptom patterns that tests do not disclose) are often considered less legitimate and are believed to have a psychiatric, unexplained, or possibly a made-up diagnosis. This common misinterpretation often leads to frustration on the part of doctors when they try to understand, diagnose, and effectively treat a condition that tests cannot identify. It erodes the patient-doctor relationship, as seen in Figure 1.

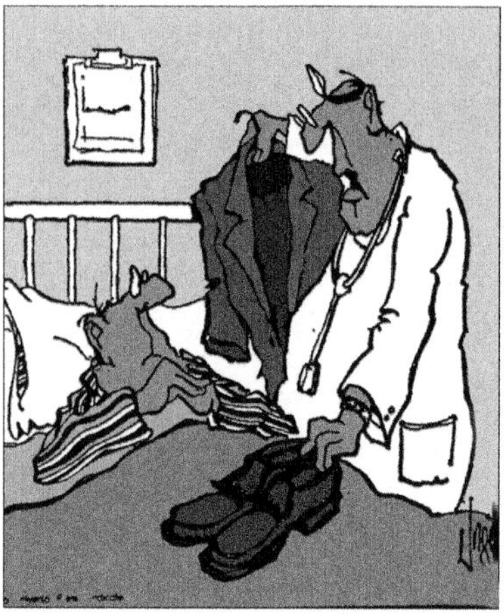

**"The results of your test were negative. Get lost!"**

**Figure 1.** Cartoon depicting a doctor's frustration working from a dualistic concept.

## Why Write This Book?

Our purpose in writing this book is to clarify how modern science replaces the antiquated dualistic model. It explains the reality of the illness experienced by patients with DGBI and the totality of the person who has it. We now know that the nerves of the brain and the GI system are physically connected and hardwired through something called the brain-gut axis. It is a fact of human physiology that the brain and GI systems are closely linked, more than any other organ system,[2] and that DGBI occur because of dysregulation of this brain-gut axis. This concept of brain-gut dysregulation is a paradigm shift in understanding that has taken place over decades of research between GI specialists and scientists from around the world. To see in a video how the brain-gut axis helps to understand the pain in IBS, click **https://romedross.video/BGAxis**.

This book is dedicated and directed to patients, but we also want it to benefit doctors who are not as familiar with DGBI. These doctors may suffer from avoidable burnout and stress because dualism adversely influences how they understand and approach patients having these disorders. Together, patients and doctors are involved in and responsible for establishing a healing relationship that serves them both. The patient with the DGBI gets better, and the doctor experiences greater understanding, leading to satisfaction with their work and their interactions with patients. This book is also for the family and friends of patients who suffer from DGBI, as well as the general public. In the end, therefore, this book is for all of us.

So let's begin.

## Ms. Byers: A Case Report

Doctors begin their training with lectures and practicums in anatomy, physiology, pharmacology, and other science-based topics. Then they need to apply this knowledge to humans and their illnesses. One way for them to learn is through case reports, which bring the application of medical knowledge within the context of the patient's illness experience.

I want to introduce you to Ms. Byers, a patient I saw many years ago. Her illness was baffling and frustrating to doctors. It was complicated because so many medical and psychological issues contributed to her illness. To understand her story requires not only medical knowledge, but also the ability to reach into her world and to learn what she experienced trying to navigate the healthcare system to feel better. I often use this case report in my lectures to illustrate how the medical system failed Ms. Byers. For our purposes, I hope it serves as an introduction to the learning that will follow.

Ms. Byers was a 33-year-old divorced woman who came to see me for chronic and severe abdominal pain, nausea, and constipation that had not responded to prior medical treatments. She said doctors never gave her a medical diagnosis, and she believed they thought it was all psychiatric. Over the years, her symptoms got worse, and she said to me assertively: "I hope you can help because everyone else has failed me." Please think of how desperate she must have felt to have to say this. Also, consider how challenging—even frightening—it would be for any doctor to take on her care.

Her story began with recurrent abdominal pain episodes at age 6, causing her to lose time at school. Later, she developed severe menstrual pain. At age 19, she went with friends to Mexico and got bacterial gastroenteritis with nausea, vomiting, fever, and diarrhea. However, unlike most cases of "Turista," all the symptoms didn't go away. Months later, she continued to have pain and diarrhea, and the doctors diagnosed irritable bowel syndrome with diarrhea (IBS-D). After that, her abdominal pain got progressively severe, her diarrhea changed to constipation, and the diagnosis became Irritable Bowel Syndrome with constipation (IBS-C). In the 5–10 years before she came to see me, the pain became more frequent and then became constant. She also developed severe migraine headaches and fibromyalgia.

Her personal life was difficult. As a young child, she had experienced many years of sexual and physical abuse from her stepfather. Her parents divorced when she was 12, and she lived with her mother, whom she felt neglected her. She left home at age 16 and became pregnant at age 17. She married the father of her child, but he also became physically and sexually abusive to her, so she and her daughter moved back to live with her mother. Ms. Byers worked as a waitress but lost her job due to work absences, and she tried to get disability.

She went to many doctors and had many tests, colonoscopies, and upper endoscopies, CT scans, pelvic ultrasound, MRIs, and a myriad of blood tests. All of them were negative. She had no insurance, and no doctor chose to provide ongoing care, so most of her treatments were in urgent clinics and emergency rooms. The doctors prescribed antispasmodics and acid blockers, which had no benefit. Some doctors prescribed antidepressants, saying it was for stress, to help her calm down. That made no sense to her.

The pain continued, and five years before she came to see me, she had had an exploratory laparotomy. The surgeons thought she might have endometriosis. She was prescribed leuprolide acetate, a hormone for endometriosis, but it was not successful. Three years before she came to see me, she had had her gallbladder removed because tests showed that her gallbladder was not functioning correctly. But its removal did not help the pain. Then, the doctors began to prescribe Percocet, an opioid narcotic, for her pain. Because it only relieved her pain temporarily, the doctors switched to Dilaudid, a more potent narcotic. At that point, her constipation got worse, and she began having bowel movements only once a week. As the pain became more severe, she required higher and higher dosages of narcotics for relief.

The interactions with her doctors were problematic. In the emergency room, she would hear them talking outside the room about her as "that problem patient." They said they wanted her to see a psychiatrist; she felt they were "blowing her off," but she knew the pain was real. Then, after a few years, the doctors began to treat her with disdain. They spoke disparagingly and refused to give her narcotic pain medication because they felt she was "drug-seeking." Ms. Byers then had no choice but to visit different emergency rooms, hoping to get relief.

When she came to my office, I found her lying on the examination table, curled up on her side with her hips flexed. She was desperate and angry. She reported severe cramping pain and nausea, saying she hadn't had a bowel movement in 2 weeks. Then she urgently requested to be hospitalized so she could get intravenous narcotic pain medication.

To watch the interview go to **https://romedross.video/2DEcCaC**.

How did we get to this point in her care? Why had it gone so poorly? To understand, we need to consider several factors:

1. Her medical diagnoses were complex and included several Disorders of Gut-Brain Interaction (DGBI), specifically: Irritable Bowel Syndrome (IBS), Opioid-Induced Constipation (OIC), Narcotic Bowel Syndrome (NBS), and Centrally Mediated Abdominal Pain Syndrome (CAPS).
2. She had overlapping psychiatric diagnoses that resulted from her earlier experiences and chronic pain. These included anxiety, depression, Post-Traumatic Stress Disorder (PTSD), and Somatic Symptom Disorder.
3. Not all doctors are familiar with the DGBI and how to treat them, nor are psychiatrists well-versed in addressing emotional difficulties in patients with these GI disorders. Furthermore, this patient, who did not understand the reason for psychological care, would not even see a psychiatrist.
4. There is a conceptual gap in understanding how this all fits together. She had

been treated unsuccessfully by doctors using a dualistic biomedical perspective. The solution is to apply biopsychosocial principles, which we will explain shortly.

5. At no time had any doctor attempted to engage with her to provide extended and ongoing care, which was something that this patient desperately needed to recover.
6. The process of her care had been brief, without clear treatment goals. It was also doctor-centered and virtually without any attention to meaningful communication. What was needed was to implement patient-centered care using effective communication skills.

See how the doctor engaged with the patient and clarified the medical issues and treatment goals at the end of the visit at **https://romedross.video/2GRui4U**.

In this book, we address all of these issues to understand better the DGBI, the patients who have them, and the best ways to diagnose and treat the patients and their illnesses. If you would like to understand the medical and psychosocial features of Ms. Byers and her illness in more detail, please click on the link to this lecture at **https://romedross.video/GersonLecture**.

As we now proceed to the rest of the book, we will follow several pathways to understand the nature of these disorders, the patients who have them, the challenges imposed on the patient and the doctor, and the solutions that benefit both.

- **Part 1** will offer the tools for learning: an explanation of the biopsychosocial model, brain-gut interactions, and patient-centered care. We will review how the concept of dualism conceptually split the mind and body into two non-interacting entities, leading to inadequate knowledge of the DGBI, ineffective treatments, and dissatisfaction on the part of both patient and doctor. I will then explain why the biopsychosocial (BPS) model is the solution to understanding and caring for patients with DGBI.
- **Part 2** catalogs all the DGBI. Because these disorders have no structural basis, we classify and diagnose them by using the innovative application of symptom-based criteria developed by the Rome Foundation. Then we discuss their treatments.
- **Part 3** offers ways to empower yourself to participate in the therapeutic process with your doctor. We describe Johannah Ruddy's experience with a DGBI to show the challenges that patients may face when patient care is ineffective. We then offer the tools to improve communication between patients and doctors to establish a positive therapeutic relationship.
- **Part 4** will help doctors (and interested patients) to understand the diagnostic and treatment process for patients having DGBI. Throughout this book, we also provide links to videos and other sources of information to enhance your learning.

Have fun.

# PART 1

# A Conceptual Understanding of the History, Philosophy, and Scientific Basis for the Disorders of Gut-Brain Interaction (DGBI)

## What Are the Disorders of Gut-Brain Interaction (DGBI)?

### *Definition*

There are 33 adult and 20 pediatric DGBI[3] in the Rome IV classification that share an underlying definition as a "group of disorders classified by gastrointestinal symptoms related to any combination of":

- Motility disturbance (abnormal movement inside the bowels)
- Visceral hypersensitivity (more intense abdominal pain than usual in response to stimuli)
- Altered mucosal and immune function (changes to the bowel's mucous membrane and immune response, e.g., "leaky gut")
- Altered gut microbiota (changes to the normal microbes found in a healthy gut, e.g., dysbiosis or imbalance of "good" and "bad" bacteria)
- Altered central nervous system (CNS) processing (changes in how the brain processes pain and other GI symptoms).

Each of the DGBI is then organized into anatomical domains, as shown in Figure 2. In this manner, irritable bowel or functional constipation would be part of the bowel disorders domain, while functional dyspepsia or nausea/vomiting syndrome would belong in the gastroduodenal disorders domain. We will elaborate on all of the DGBI diagnoses later so you will understand what you may have and why. Just having this knowledge can have therapeutic value.

### *Putting the DGBI on the Map: The Role of the Rome Foundation*

How did we come to understand DGBI? At the turn of the 19th century, abdominal pain, diarrhea, nausea, or vomiting were considered merely a collection of symptoms. From the 1950s well into the 1980s, structural disorders, like peptic ulcer, GI tumors, diverticulitis, pancreatic disease, and inflammatory bowel disease (IBD –

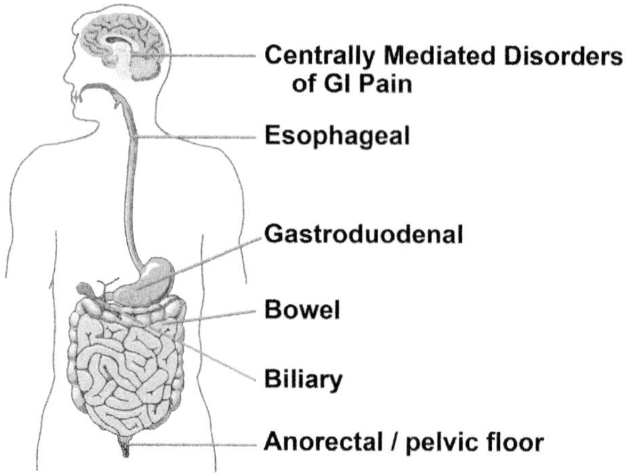


**Figure 2.** The anatomical basis we use to categorize DGBI according to the Rome IV classification. This diagram shows the anatomic domains of the GI system that Rome IV uses to organize the DGBI. Each DGBI diagnosis is placed into one of these domains. Thus, IBS and functional constipation are bowel disorders, and functional dyspepsia or nausea/vomiting syndromes are gastroduodenal disorders.

ulcerative colitis and Crohn's disease) dominated the field of gastroenterology. They were easy to diagnose using imaging methods like x-rays and later endoscopies. Yet these structural diagnoses applied to only about half of the patients seen in GI clinics. The other half had symptoms not diagnosed by imaging studies, which were called "functional." At the time, clinicians and scientists attributed these functional symptoms to abnormal movements of the GI tract and called them motility disorders, which relates to how rapidly or slowly the intestines move their contents along. Motility testing can help to make some diagnoses like gastroparesis (delayed emptying of stomach contents) or esophageal motility disorders (e.g., achalasia, diffuse esophageal spasm). It can also demonstrate the physiological basis for some symptoms, like diarrhea or constipation (i.e., the intestines moving too fast or too slow). Still, these tests cannot diagnose them, though they are useful for research. Notably, however, motility testing does not diagnose all the common GI symptoms like pain, bloating, or nausea. Agencies like the National Institutes of Health (NIH) and the Food and Drug Administration (FDA), therefore, had no basis for diagnosing and characterizing these symptoms, which left pharmaceutical companies with no practical way to identify these patients to study in clinical trials. By the 1980s, there seemed to be no solution.

A major enhancement toward understanding these disorders occurred with the creation of the Rome Foundation, an international nonprofit 501(c)3 organization (www.theromefoundation.org), whose mission is "To help patients with Disorders of Gut-Brain Interaction." This organization introduced the concept of identifying, classifying, characterizing, and treating the symptoms that patients brought to their doctors. The Foundation developed symptom-based criteria to diagnose these disorders since imaging and motility testing had failed.

I founded the Rome Foundation some 30 years ago and currently serve as President Emeritus and Chief of Operations. At that time, I was part of an international collaboration with W. Grant Thompson, MD (Canada), William Whitehead, PhD (USA), Nicholas Talley, MD, MPH (Australia), and Enrico Corazziari, MD (Italy), and these notables have continued to distinguish themselves in the field. We came together as doctors and scientists who understood that the many patients we were treating who were then called "functional" did not exist within a conceptual framework. According to the dualistic understanding of the time, they had no "disease." We believed that creating a classification system for the functional GI disorders (later to be called DGBI) would "put them on the map," so to speak. Then patients could be identified and studied scientifically—and, in the process, be legitimized.

We began with each of us conducting our own clinical and epidemiological research. Then, by finding the commonalities, we worked together through collaboration and consensus. The first study was the 1978 creation of the Manning Criteria, a group of symptoms to diagnose irritable bowel syndrome (IBS).[4] Developing criteria was a complete departure from other research, which used disease-based or physiological measures to make diagnoses.[5] The authors surveyed 32 patients previously diagnosed by doctors to have IBS and 33 patients with organic disease. They gave them a questionnaire with 15 symptoms thought typical of irritable bowel syndrome (IBS) to see if any of these items distinguished the two groups. Four symptoms were significantly more common in the IBS patient group: distension of the belly, relief of pain with bowel movement, and looser and more frequent bowel movements with the onset of pain. The more of these symptoms that were present, the more likely it was that the patient had IBS. Concurrently, the rest of us were doing clinical and epidemiological studies, and we arrived at similar observations. Our studies were similar and mutually supportive and that offered greater confidence to use collections of symptoms to make a diagnosis.

In 1987, a working team of five international GI experts from different countries including Dr. Thompson and myself created a consensus document on diagnostic criteria for IBS and presented it at Roma 88, The International Congress of Gastroenterology, under Dr. Aldo Torsoli who was the president. This document, published in 1989, was the first to establish the idea of using a team of experts to create diagnostic criteria by consensus.[6] The next step was to bring the doctors together to establish guidelines for the classification and diagnosis for all the DGBI.

By the late 1980s, many papers were starting to appear on other functional GI disorders like functional dyspepsia, functional heartburn, or post-cholecystectomy biliary pain. However, no one had figured out a viable way to characterize and diagnose these disorders systematically. To this end, my collaborators and I created a working team to publish a classification system for all the functional GI disor-

| | "Organic" GI disorder | Motility disorder | Disorders of Gut-Brain Interaction |
|---|---|---|---|
| Primary domain | Organ morphology | Organ function | Illness experience |
| Criterion | **Pathology (disease)** | **Altered motility** | **Symptoms** |
| Measurement | Histology<br>Pathology<br>Endoscopy<br>Radiology | Motility<br>Visceral sensitivity | Motility<br>Visceral sensitivity<br>Symptom criteria (Rome)<br>Psychometric |
| Treatment options | **Medications**<br>**Surgery**<br>**Ther. endoscopy** | **Pro / anti-kinetics**<br>**Surgery**<br>**Pacing / Stimulator** | **Pro / anti-kinetics**<br>**Neuromodulators**<br>**Behavioral** |
| Examples | Esophagitis<br>Peptic ulcer<br>IBD<br>Colon cancer | Diffuse esoph. spasm<br>Gastroparesis<br>Pseudo-obstruction<br>Colonic inertia | Esophageal chest pain<br>Functional dyspepsia<br>IBS<br>Centrally mediated abdominal pain |

**Figure 3.** Categorization of gastrointestinal disorders. Pathological or structural abnormalities characterize the "organic" disorders, while motility testing defines the motility disorders, and the use of symptom-based criteria diagnoses the Disorders of Gut-Brain Interaction (DGBI). See text for details.

ders.[7] The use of consensus to classify the diagnostic criteria for these disorders changed the way doctors diagnosed these patients, and more and more research used symptom-based criteria to identify study subjects. Then the Food and Drug Administration (FDA) and other regulatory agencies, as well as the pharmaceutical industry, saw the value of these criteria and applied them when conducting clinical research on patients. This work led to the creation of the Rome Foundation (**https://romedross.video/origins**).

Figure 3 shows the organization of gastrointestinal disorders. As noted, the "organic" disorders are structurally based. In contrast, disturbances in pressures generated in the bowel using motility testing identify the motility disorders. Finally, the DGBI use symptom-based diagnostic criteria for diagnosis. So now, these disorders are "on the map," not being just a collection of symptoms and thus are legitimized (**https://romedross.video/accomplishments**).

By 1990, the Rome Foundation's symptom-based criteria became entrenched as the basis for identifying, defining, and classifying the DGBI. The classification system changed the landscape of GI medicine and opened the door to highly sophisticated research to help understand and treat a large variety of DGBI. It also created an entirely new comprehension, breaking through dualistic thinking and legitimizing DGBI to patients and their providers. Figure 4 traces the evolution of medical research from early physiological studies in the 1950s to the present. The

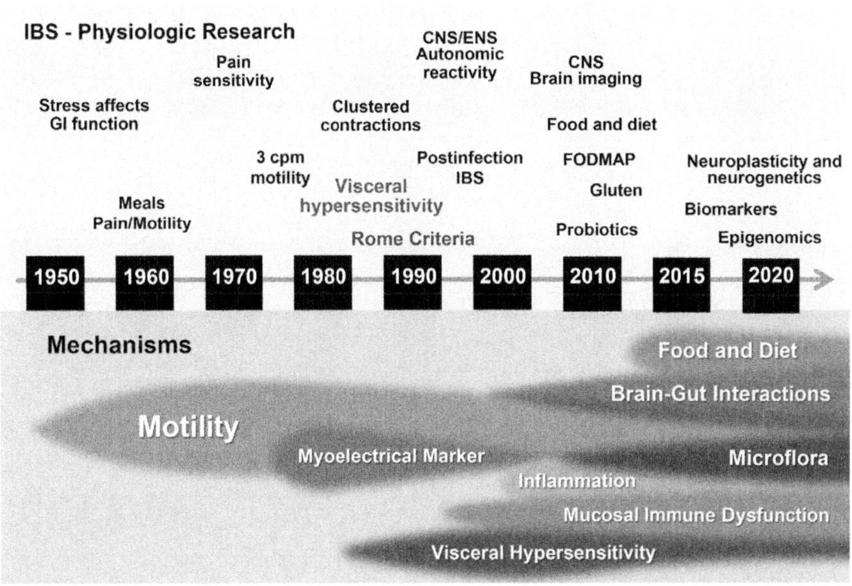


**Figure 4.** History of physiological research on IBS and FGID. This timeline shows some of the critical research studies on the top and the research domains on the bottom. From 1950 until 1990, research focused on motility. After 1990, and with the emergence of the Rome criteria to diagnose and categorize these patients, new research began. This led to the discovery of other physiological factors to explain these disorders: visceral hypersensitivity (increased sensitivity of the bowel) and then to studies on brain-gut interactions, inflammation, microflora, and the role of food and diet. The Rome classification system and criteria enabled the identification of patients for research.

use of this symptom-based (Rome) criteria, beginning in 1990, led to an explosion of diverse areas of research and our current understanding of the DGBI.

The Rome Foundation has continued to grow. Members collaborate to review the evolving science in the field every 6–10 years. Since the 1990s, the Rome Foundation has updated its books from Rome I (1994), II (2000), III (2006), and IV (2016). Rome V has just begun and will be completed in 2026. These publications include new knowledge and guidelines to help clinicians understand and manage DGBI. One principal recommendation for Rome IV, in 2016, was to change the terminology from Functional GI Disorders (or FGID) to DGBI as we became more aware that "functional" implied illegitimacy and was stigmatizing to patients. As new science emerges in the field, the Rome Foundation continues to modify its diagnostic and treatment guidelines.

## What Is Mind-Body Dualism and How Has It Affected Medical Practice?

Now that we have learned how the term DGBI came about, let's understand why patients who have them have very different healthcare experiences than patients who have a peptic ulcer, IBD, or other structurally based diseases. A few years ago, over one month, I listed the statements that patients with DGBI said to me during their first clinical visit:

"Doctors don't believe me."
"There MUST be something wrong."
"I know it's real."
"I just want you to open me up and find out the problem."
"You don't think it's in my head, do you?"
"Sometimes, I feel like I'm going crazy."
"Nobody knows what I'm going through."
"I feel like I'm not the person I used to be."
"I feel so alone with this."
"I feel like such a burden to my family."
"I have no control over this."
"I feel I may have caused some damage."
"I feel like a failure."
"I feel ashamed."

As you look down the list, you see a deepening sense of distress, ranging from not being believed to fearing that the symptoms are not legitimate or are even psychiatric, to feeling isolation, loneliness, lack of control, self-blame, and even shame. In my experience, most patients with a DGBI want more than diagnosis and treatment; they also want to be believed and to have their symptoms validated.

I encourage you to look at this list, take a step back, and consider: Why is this happening?

To address this question, we need to go back in history to the origins and the influence, over centuries, of the biomedical model and mind-body dualism on health care. Then we can understand how it became clear that this system was detrimental to patients and doctors. The failure of the biomedical model to explain illness provided the right environment for the emergence of the biopsychosocial model since it led to the scientific understanding of DGBI and the path to an effective healthcare solution (**https://romedross.video/MDLivePPR**).

### *The Evolution of Dualistic Thinking in Western Civilization*

*"The concept of the separation of mind and body is dominant and pervasive in Western thinking.... The consequence of that is that symptoms that have no morphologic [structural] basis are not amenable to study and are not understood. This has had profound negative effects on research, patient care, and the patient-doctor relationship."*—Douglas A. Drossman, MD

**https://romedross.video/12Gurus**

Since the beginning of recorded medical history, the concept of illness and disease has fluctuated over time and across cultures between a unified, holistic approach (which later evolved as the biopsychosocial model) and a dualistic approach. Within Western civilization, *holism* was first advanced over 2,000 years ago by Plato, and then by Aristotle and Hippocrates in ancient Greece. Plato stated (400 BCE): *"The greatest mistake in the treatment of diseases is that there are physicians for the body and physicians for the soul, although the two cannot be separated."* This approach accepts medical symptoms and behavioral disturbances as legitimate features of the individual and their illness. It has traditionally existed in early Western writings and currently lives in Eastern cultures.[8]

Mind-body dualism gradually evolved throughout Western Europe with the dominance of Christianity. It became entrenched in 1637 when the French philosopher René Descartes proposed that the *"material like body"* and the *"thinking mind"*[2] were distinct and separate entities. This concept, known as Cartesian dualism, aligned with sociocultural influences of the time, relating to the separation of church and state. It rapidly became the prevailing view, profoundly influencing the conceptualization and treatment of medical disease. Before that time, church doctrine held that the spirit resided within the body—that body and spirit were not separate—so, it was not permitted to perform human dissection or surgery. However, Descartes' ideas "lifted" the mind and soul from the body.

With the acceptance that the two were separate, human dissection could now be done, leading to the ability to observe the body and its organs visually. Therefore, medical diagnosis evolved to be based on abnormalities of structure, leading to diagnosing diseases like ulcers or cancer. Abnormalities of structure then led to the emergence of the scientific fields of pathology and histology, readily discernable, and microscopic vehicles for the detection of disease. Over time, new tests (e.g., x-rays, CT scans, MRI imaging) developed to detect more specific and elaborate structural abnormalities in the body.

These imaging methods brought to light new knowledge of diseases and their diagnoses and treatments. But what if there was "illness without disease"? The ability to test and see led to medical understanding in strictly morphological terms. It also, at the time, led to considering mental illness as unfit for scientific study, since it aligned with alteration of the spirit. Initially, spiritual possession—and later, insanity—were thought to explain illness and human behaviors when there was no structural basis. As a result, non-structurally based symptoms and behaviors came to be considered illegitimate, and people who had them were stigmatized. These patients were sent to asylums and deemed not amenable to medical study. In the 19th century, Benjamin Rush, an American doctor, politician, and educator, conceived bringing the study of mental illness into medical schools. Because mind-body dualism was so entrenched in health care, however, this did not occur until early in the 20th century.

### *The Effect on Modern Health Care*

Now, let's move forward four centuries to the present. When a patient in the 21st century reports symptoms and diagnostic studies repeatedly do not show that anything is wrong, what happens? For patients and doctors, mind-body dualism says whatever *is* wrong is not real or belongs strictly to the brain—is a psychiatric disorder (i.e., "in your head.") Therefore, in Western culture (but not in Eastern cultures, where Descartes had no influence), it is more credible to have a structurally based disease. Structurally based diseases are considered legitimate due to the biomedical model and mind-body dualism. Now we can understand why patients with functional illnesses like DGBI often have a different experience with doctors than do patients with a structural issue. In addition to considering structural abnormalities the only basis of legitimate disease, the concept of Cartesian reductionism asserted that there is only a single cause of any illness. This single cause is considered necessary for the disease to exist and sufficient to explain how it presents itself in everyone. It is supposed to explain not only the illness experience but all its consequences. The incorrect presumption is that some biological susceptibility or predisposition (such as the presence of a specific gene), when combined with an environmental event (such as an infection), will trigger a disease. Based on this model, the disease may have psychological effects, but these effects do not in any way influence the biological nature of the disease. If you would like more information on the historical aspects of these models, go to **https://romedross.video/12Gurus**.

Biomedical reductionism—in other words, the single-cause theory—can be useful for some acute diseases, such as a bacterial infection. But what about chronic illness? This model does not account for the variability in how patients experience chronic diseases like diabetes or cancer. For example, why would one person with a peptic ulcer have no pain until they have a perforation or an obstruction? In contrast, another one has a lot of pain and goes to the doctor's time and again, though endoscopic studies show only minimal or no inflammation. What do doctors do when a patient presents with illness but no disease? They may repeatedly focus on trying to find an underlying disease, to no avail.

The failure of this biomedical and dualistic model has behavioral consequences. Patients seeking a structural diagnosis go to doctors who initially engage with them to find a structural disease. When not found, patients may intensify their request or

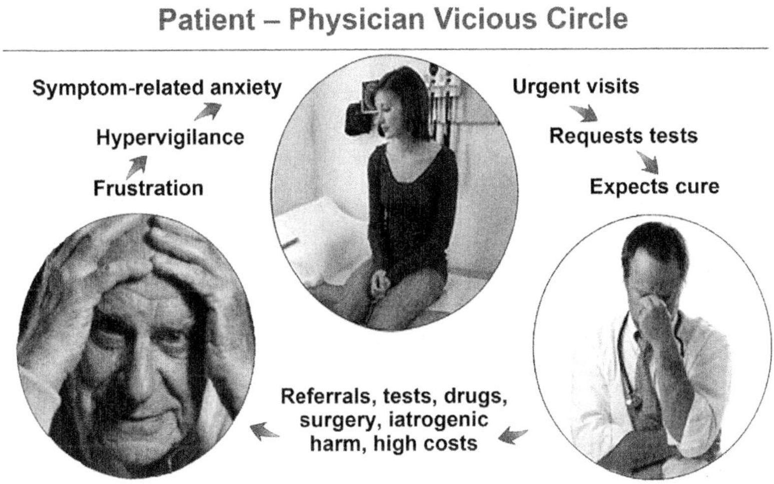


**Figure 5.** The vicious cycle of dissatisfaction using a dualistic approach to DGBI. This figure illustrates the negative cycle of frustration between patients and doctors who adhere to a dualistic model of illness and disease, and when the brain-gut axis is not understood. The patient makes urgent requests for testing and diagnosis. The doctor, in turn, keeps trying to find out what is wrong, using their usual arsenal of referrals, tests, drugs, surgery, etc. This only results in high costs and may even be harmful to the patient. The patient then develops heightened anxiety about their non-diagnosed symptoms and becomes hypervigilant to them. They experience mounting frustration and concern and continue to make requests for more tests, all in the pursuit of finding a cure. This vicious cycle of dissatisfaction is destructive to patients and doctors and leads to no solution.

seek care with other doctors. In turn, doctors keep trying, but when they don't see a disease, they become frustrated, defensive, and angry; they may withdraw from the process or refer the patient elsewhere,[1] which may negatively affect patient safety and the clinical outcome. This scenario sets up a vicious cycle of dissatisfaction between patient and doctor, as we show in Figure 5.

Our central point is that real understanding and effective treatment of people with DGBI require doctors to recognize that these are multi-determined disorders that employ two-way communication between the gut and the brain and with psychosocial consequences. The doctor needs to acknowledge the reality of the patient's complaint, make a diagnosis based on Rome criteria, provide empathy, and engage in a patient-centered interaction, addressing not only the patient's symptoms, but also the psychosocial issues that accompany them, to detach from the vicious cycle of dissatisfaction shown above. When this occurs, it is my experience that patients accept the diagnosis, become a partner in their care, and ultimately reduce their search for other diagnoses.

You may feel that there must always be a structural basis for symptoms, but that is often not the case, and it is undoubtedly not for DGBI. Even if a test discloses an

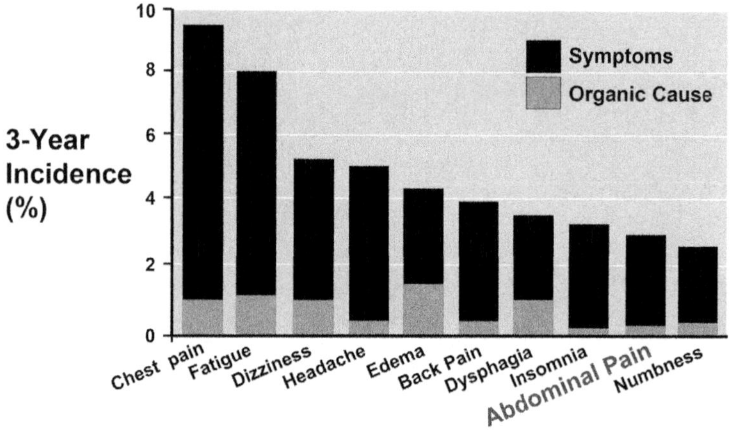


**Figure 6.** The proportion of patients presenting with symptoms vs. organic causes eventually identified. This figure shows the results of Dr. Kroenke's 3-year clinical study to determine the proportion of patients who presented with symptoms (shown in blue) as opposed to organic causes (shown in orange). In every category, the organic disease occurred in only a small proportion of the illness presentations. From Kroenke K, Mangelsdorff AD. Common symptoms in ambulatory care: Incidence, evaluation, therapy and outcome. Am J Med 1989;86:262–266.

anatomic finding, it may not explain the illness. Figure 6 demonstrates a clinical study by Dr. Kurt Kroenke, who evaluated patients seen at a primary-care clinic over a 3-year period that presented with the most common medical illnesses. Of the top ten symptoms seen, a structural diagnosis was eventually identified in only about 10%.[9] So while the biomedical model focuses on doctors learning to diagnose disease, the vast majority of patients have illness without disease.

### *Dealing with Uncertainty Is Difficult for Doctors*

It is no surprise, following from the above, that when Renee Fox, PhD, a medical sociologist, studied medical student experience, attitudes, and behaviors in the 1950s,[10] she found that one of their most significant challenges was dealing with the uncertainties seen in clinical practice. Students found it very difficult to deal with symptoms not explained by structural abnormalities as with DGBI, since their training was about medical disease.

The legacy of mind-body dualism has left Western medicine with the notion (as shown in Figure 7) that disease is dominant, with its valid, structural abnormalities, and doctors call that organic. Less well understood and down the ladder of importance is an illness—the *perception* of ill health—and that is called functional. Doctors may feel uncertain about a patient's illness when it is not anchored in structure. Yet illness is genuine to the person who experiences it, even when others may not believe it. Elaine Scarry, who wrote in her book, *The Body in Pain,* that *"to have pain is to have certainty; to hear that another person has pain is to have doubt."*[11]

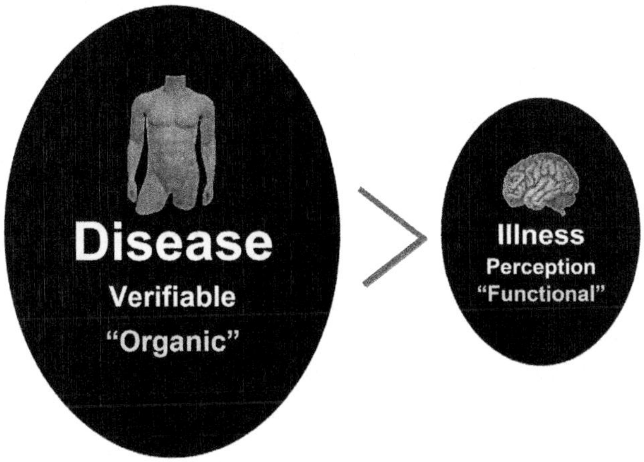


**Figure 7.** Comparative value placed upon organic disease vs. functional illness. This figure illustrates how—because the brain-gut axis is not understood and accepted—verifiable disease is considered valid while functional illness is diminished.

## What Is the Biopsychosocial Model and Why Do We Need It?

My mentor, George Engel, MD (see Figure 8), first coined this term in his seminal publication in the prestigious journal, *Science,* in 1977.[12] He noted that: *"The dominant biomedical model of disease leaves no room within its framework for the social, psychological and behavioral dimensions of illness."* He then went on to say: *"A biopsychosocial model is proposed that provides a blueprint for research, a framework for teaching and a design for action in the real world of health care."* This presentation by Dr. Engel filmed over 30 years ago demonstrates the nature and value of the biopsychosocial model in clinical care (**https://romedross.video/Engel**).

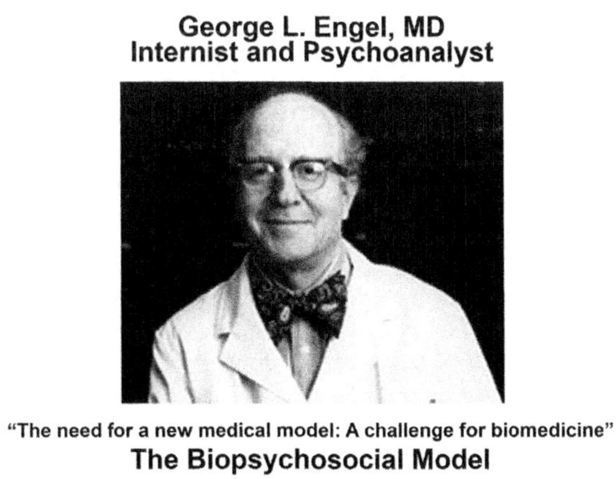


**Figure 8.** George L. Engel, MD, my mentor, was an internist and psychoanalyst who first coined the term *biopsychosocial model.*

These prophetic words lay bare and overcome the deficits of dualistic thinking in medicine. Biopsychosocial is a big word, but the basic idea is that the brain and the body interact and influence each other. *Bio*, the first part of the name, is short for biological; *psycho* refers to the psychological or mental component that affects our bodies; and *social* refers to the social aspects of our lives, including family, friends, and other environmental factors that play a role in DGBI.

Because we have learned that the brain and gut interact physiologically through the "brain-gut axis," we must keep this reciprocal interaction front and center in the way we view and treat DGBI. Calm the brain, and you calm the gut; calm the gut, and you calm the brain. This need to treat DGBI as a two-way street is our challenge in understanding and successfully treating people with these disorders. The biopsychosocial approach acknowledges and incorporates a role for these psychosocial factors in illness and disease, and vice versa.

### *Making Sense of the Biopsychosocial Model*

Below, we show and explain this biopsychosocial model (Figure 9), which has provided the operational basis for my research and teaching[13] and for collaboration within the Rome Foundation.[3]

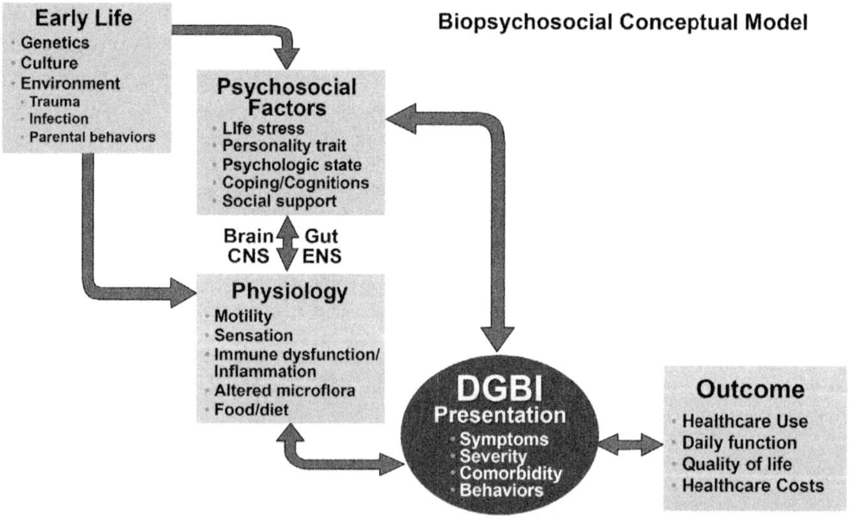


**Figure 9.** The Biopsychosocial Conceptual Model for DGBI. This figure shows what predetermines a DGBI, the early-life predisposing influences, the brain-gut reciprocating factors that come into play in these disorders, and their outcome, affecting daily activities and health care in general. Thus, a DGBI is the product of these interactions between psychosocial factors and physiological changes to the gut via the brain-gut axis. From Drossman DA, Functional Gastrointestinal Disorders and the Rome IV Process. In: Drossman DA, Chang L, Chey WD, et al. Rome IV Functional Gastrointestinal Disorders - Disorders of Gut-Brain Interaction. 4th ed. Raleigh, NC: Rome Foundation.

Ever wonder why some people get sicker than others, even though they have the same diagnosis? The biopsychosocial model helps explain the variability of human illness based on the many factors shown here. As shown in Figure 9, early-life factors (left side of diagram), genetics, sociocultural influences, and the environment can affect our development of personality traits, susceptibility to life stresses, our psychological state, how we think, and our coping skills. These factors also influence our susceptibility to dysfunctions in the gut: abnormal sensitivity or motility, inflammation of the mucous membrane or dysregulation of its immune functions, changes in the healthy gut microbial environment, and the effect that food and nutritional substances can have on it. Does this sound familiar? It's the definition of the DGBI.

On top of that, this "brain-gut" connection allows for each organ system to have reciprocal influences. Emotional states affect motility, sensation, and even immunity in the gut; conversely, pain and motility disturbances lead to emotional distress, anxiety, and even depression. It's a two-way street. The combination of these effects leads to the experience of illness and the symptoms and patient behaviors that result.

The biopsychosocial model also proposes a hierarchical relationship that affects the order of biological systems, from the microscopic levels to society (Figure 10). Illness and disease result from simultaneously interacting systems at the cellular, tissue, organismal, interpersonal, and environmental levels. The model integrates

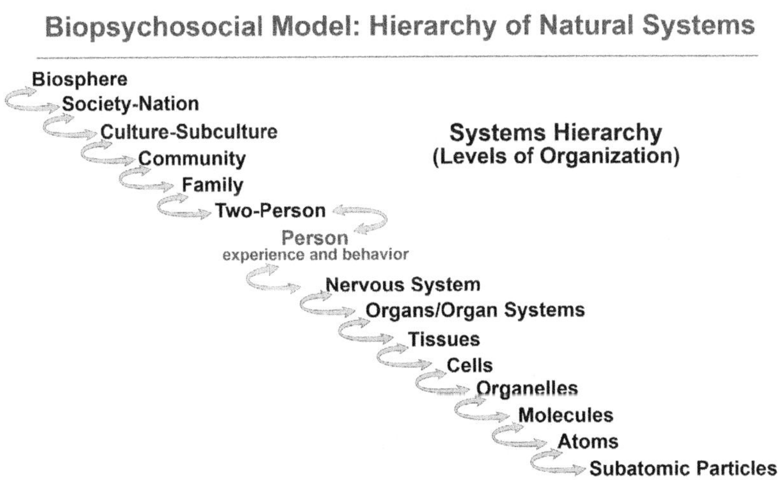


**Figure 10.** The biopsychosocial model describes a hierarchy of interrelated biological systems that exist in a continuum. Every unit in this system is a whole and a part of the other systems to which it is related. For example, coronavirus infection affects tissues or cells, and this impacts on the person and society. Conversely, societal change, such as a change in health policy, for example to wear a mask to contain viral exposure, will affect the individual and likelihood of infection. Another example—dysbiosis in the gut—will influence the development of IBS. It will also alter the individual's emotional state; conversely, emotional distress can change the body's regulation of bacteria in the gut (see below). From Engel GL. The clinical application of the Biopsychosocial Model. 1980 Am J Psychiatry, 137:535–544.

biological science with the unique features of the individual and determines the degree to which biological and psychosocial factors interact to explain their disease, illness, and outcome. Even the most sophisticated diagnostic techniques are not sufficient to explain the degree, variability, or even the presence of some GI symptoms, or the patient's experience and behavior related to them. The biopsychosocial model explains these complex relationships.[5, 13]

The biopsychosocial model provides the template for the development of DGBI vis-à-vis interaction of the gut and the brain. Let's see how this plays out in a common GI disorder. We use Figure 11 to show how a gastrointestinal infection, in association with stressful experiences such as trauma or a significant loss, enables the development of post-infection IBS.

The biopsychosocial model not only explains how psychosocial factors and biological events cause DGBI, it also allows doctors to respond in various ways, based on the uniqueness of the individual. So, looking again at Figure 9, a more limited bacterial gastroenteritis that develops in a person who has no concurrent psychosocial difficulties and excellent coping skills may not develop into IBS, or

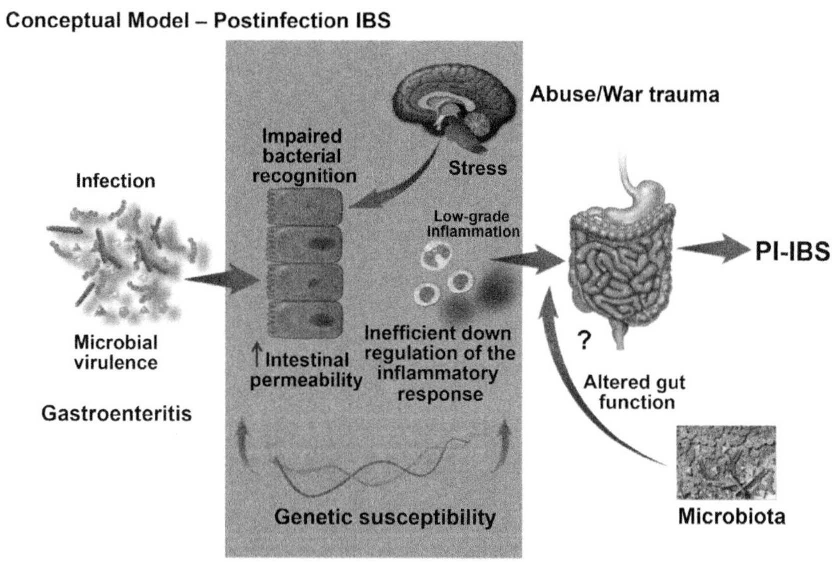


**Figure 11.** How post-infection IBS can develop. This figure illustrates what happens when an infection weakens the lining of the bowel (some people call it "leaky gut"), compromising the integrity of the bowel wall, and bacteria and toxins leak in. When this happens in combination with stressors, such as abuse, it amplifies the degree of impaired immunity by causing increased nerve sensitivity (visceral hypersensitivity), which produces pain and diarrhea consistent with IBS. This type of IBS is called post-infection IBS. From Collins SM et al. Postinfectious chronic gut dysfunction. From bench to bedside. Am J Gastroenterol Suppl 2012;1:2–8.

if IBS does develop, it may be mild. That person may not even seek medical care. On the other hand, an individual with a more severe infection, who is living with difficult psychosocial conditions, high life stress, a history of abuse, or ineffective coping skills, is more likely to develop severe IBS, go to the doctor frequently, get little relief, and have a more unsatisfactory outcome.

We can extend the biopsychosocial model beyond the individual to interpersonal and familial influences on illness. A family that displays overconcern about their child's illness, or interprets specific symptoms as a threat and approaches doctors with anxiety and worry, may intensify the patient's symptoms, lead to more doctor visits, and even to more illness behaviors later in life.[14] Conversely, a family that diminishes the patient's distress (tells them to "suck it up") may lead the patient to feel emotionally isolated and unheard. Also, the latter approach may lessen the patient's ability to justifiably represent themselves to their doctors later in life ("I don't want to bother you but..."). See Johannah Ruddy's experience of this in Part 3. However, a family that appropriately adapts and responds to the child's illness and psychosocial concerns, and provides appropriate support, will reduce the impact of the patient's illness experience and lead to more healthy illness behaviors later in life.

### *How the Biopsychosocial Model and the Use of Symptom-Based Criteria Help to Remedy the Challenges Doctors Face in Treating DGBI*

With this new understanding, we can begin to remedy some of the challenges that doctors face if they adhere to a dualistic model when treating patients with DGBI.

Because doctors are under pressure to see more patients in less time, they may feel compelled to order expensive and often unnecessary tests. Some may also prioritize their time to focus on patients whom they perceive as sicker or as having "real" disease. However, with DGBI, it is the data obtained from the medical history, rather than testing alone, that leads to a proper diagnosis and a plan of care. Confidence in using symptom-based criteria reduces the need for testing "to rule out organic disease." With DGBI, too much reliance on technology can be ineffective and misleading.[1] Furthermore, learning excellent communication skills allows for interpersonal engagement that is mutually gratifying. When patients like doctors, doctors like patients.

Also, the qualitative aspects of patient care, such as taking a complete medical history, conducting a physical exam, and sitting with the patient and listening to them, are disappearing from office visits, often replaced by doctors staring at computer screens and clicking boxes. Unfortunately, physicians are increasingly required to handle more and more administrative duties and attend to licensing and certification concerns that take time from their patients. This may cause them to disengage from their patients during visits and shift their attention to non-medical and impersonal tasks. Likewise, doctors' understanding of the positive consequences of practical communication skills is often scant, and they may have had little if any training in such skills.[1] However, when doctors learn to engage, listen, and base their judgments for diagnosis and treatment on the patient's needs, expectations, and psychosocial milieu (patient-centered care), the illness is better understood and more appropriately treated. This is what we discuss in Part 3.

Furthermore, the Rome Foundation in collaboration with DrossmanCare has committed to teaching doctors communication skills to help them develop a bio-psychosocial approach to the care of patients with DGBI, and later in this book, we offer you some of these skills for your own use when seeing your doctor. For further information, go to **https://romedross.video/2kfU3Dd**.

## PART 2

# The Disorders of Gut-Brain Interaction (DGBI)

NOW WE ARE READY to list and explain all the adult DGBI, based on the most recent Rome IV classification.[3, 15] First, we provide in Table 1 all the adult DGBI, categorized by their main domains: esophageal, gastroduodenal, bowel, centrally mediated, gallbladder and biliary, and anorectal. Then we list the pediatric DGBI, categorized by neonate/toddler (0–4) and child/adolescent (5 and older) domains. Following this, we go into more detail about all the adult DGBI, including their definition, their pathophysiology (what is causing the symptoms), the clinical evaluation (how doctors diagnose) including the Rome IV criteria, and the treatments. Finally, we offer an appendix that lists all the Rome IV criteria, as well as a glossary of terms to aid in understanding.

There are two caveats to consider:

***First, diagnostic studies and treatments, including dosages of drugs, are recommended from the medical literature and my clinical experience. For the most part, these recommendations conform to the practices of gastroenterologists working in the field of DGBI. Some of the treatments are considered "off label," meaning that they are not necessarily approved by the FDA for the condition discussed but have shown benefit in the scientific literature. Further, the recommendations I have made are done so in general for these disorders and may not specifically apply to your clinical situation. The recommendations are a guide for you to learn about these treatments and to discuss them with your doctor.***

***Second, unless otherwise indicated, diagnosing a DGBI by Rome IV criteria requires that the symptoms described must have begun at least 6 months before the diagnosis is made and then must meet full Rome diagnostic criteria for at least 3 months. We require this to eliminate short-lived symptoms (e.g., acute gastroenteritis or discomforts from overeating) that may occur from time to time. Those are common symptoms that would not warrant a DGBI diagnosis.***

*Table 1. DGBI Classified by Rome IV (see Appendix A for full criteria)*

| A. Esophageal Disorders[16] | |
|---|---|
| **Functional Disorder** | **Functional definition and links to more information** |
| **A1. Functional Chest Pain** | Recurring, unexplained chest pain behind the sternum that is not experienced as heartburn but is believed to be related to the esophagus. Heart disease should be excluded by medical evaluation or cardiac diagnostic studies. |
| **A2. Functional Heartburn** | Burning discomfort or pain that is experienced behind the breastbone (retrosternal) that does not respond to acid-blocking treatments and is not caused by increased acid reflux or any structural diagnosis or motility disorder. |
| **A3. Reflux Hypersensitivity** | Heartburn or chest pain when endoscopy and pH studies are normal, but symptoms occur when acid enters the esophagus. Esophageal PH testing shows no increased acid, but the esophagus is found to be sensitive to acid. **https://romedross.video/2FtbM1H** |
| **A4. Globus** | Persistent or intermittent non-painful sensation of having a lump or foreign body in the throat. It occurs episodically and is located in the midline above the sternal notch. |
| **A5. Functional Dysphagia** | Sense of solid or liquid foods sticking, lodging, or passing abnormally through the esophagus. **https://romedross.video/2M8N5ez** |

| B. Gastroduodenal Disorders[17] | |
|---|---|
| **Functional Disorder** | **Functional definition and links to more information** |
| **B1. Functional Dyspepsia** | Any of the following apply: (1) The unpleasant sensation of food staying in the stomach after a meal ("postprandial fullness"); (2) the unpleasant feeling that the stomach is overfilled soon after starting to eat ("early satiety"); (3) subjective, intense pain in the area just above the stomach ("epigastric pain") and/or (4) unpleasant, subjective sensation of heat in the epigastrium. These symptoms significantly impact usual activities. There are two subtypes of functional dyspepsia, as shown below in B1a and B1b. They may overlap. **https://romedross.video/36uTGaA** |
| **-B1a. Postprandial Distress Syndrome (PDS)** | Uncomfortable sensation of being too full soon after eating a meal or becoming full so early that eating a regular-sized meal is prevented. PDS is characterized exclusively by meal-induced symptoms. |

*continues*

| B. Gastroduodenal Disorders[17] | |
|---|---|
| **Functional Disorder** | **Functional definition and links to more information** |
| **-B1b. Epigastric Pain Syndrome (EPS)** | Epigastric pain or burning that does not occur exclusively after meals, may occur during fasting, and may be improved or worsened by food. |
| **B2. Belching Disorders** | The audible escape of air from the esophagus or the stomach into the pharynx. This is only considered a disorder when it is excessive and becomes troublesome. Belching disorders are sub-classified into gastric belching or supragastric belching, described below in B2a and B2b. |
| **-B2a. Excessive Supra-gastric Belching (from esophagus)** | Excessive belching that occurs more than 3 days a week, caused by gas that originates from the esophagus. See B2, above, for a fuller description. |
| **-B2b. Excessive Gastric Belching (from stomach)** | Excessive belching that occurs more than 3 days a week, caused by gas that originates from the stomach. See B2, above, for a fuller description. |
| **B3. Nausea and Vomiting Disorder** | Nausea is the unpleasant sensation of needing to vomit, typically felt in the upper abdomen immediately above the stomach, or in the throat (see B3a below). Vomiting is the forceful oral expulsion of gastrointestinal contents associated with contraction of the abdominal and chest wall muscles (see B3b below). **http://bit.ly/2wW5hiD** |
| **-B3a. Chronic Nausea Vomiting Syndrome (CNVS)** | Nausea occurring at least one day a week that is severe enough to impact usual activities, and/or one or more vomiting episodes a week. Eating disorders and self-induced vomiting must be excluded, and tests (including an upper endoscopy) find no evidence of organic abnormality. **http://bit.ly/2wW5hiD** |
| **-B3b. Cyclic Vomiting Syndrome (CVS)** | Intermittent stereotypical episodes of intense vomiting (up to 30 times a day) that may occur multiple times a year, lasting for a week or more, and the absence of nausea and vomiting between episodes. **http://bit.ly/2wW5hiD** |
| **-B3c. Cannabinoid Hyperemesis Syndrome (CHS)** | Episodes of vomiting similar to CVS in their onset, duration, and frequency, but they occur after prolonged, excessive cannabis use and stop when cannabis use is discontinued. **https://romedross.video/2FtbM1H** |
| **B4. Rumination Syndrome** | Repetitive, effortless regurgitation of recently eaten food into the mouth, which is then re-swallowed or spit out. Regurgitation is not preceded by retching and occurs before the food has turned into acid. **https://theromefoundation.org/q-a-rumination-2/** |

| C. Bowel Disorders[18] | |
|---|---|
| **Functional Disorder** | **Functional definition and links to more information** |
| **C1. Irritable Bowel Syndrome (IBS)** | A bowel disorder in which recurrent abdominal pain is related to defecation and associated with constipation, diarrhea, or a mixture of both; abdominal bloating and distension may also be present. The IBS subtypes C, D, M, and U are differentiated by relative proportions of the stool form, as discussed below. **https://romedross.video/Q_A_IBSCD** |
| **–IBS with Predominant Constipation (IBS-C)** | IBS with more than one-fourth (25%) of bowel movements that are hard or lumpy (Types 1 and 2 on Bristol Stool Form Scale – BSFS). **https://romedross.video/2NrTXVe** |
| **–IBS with Predominant Diarrhea (IBS-D)** | IBS with more than one-fourth (25%) of bowel movements that are loose or watery (Types 6 and 7 on BSFS) **https://romedross.video/2GJIEnt** |
| **–IBS with Mixed Bowel Habits (IBS-M)** | IBS with a mixture of hard/lumpy and loose/watery bowel movements, each more than one-fourth (25%) of bowel movements. |
| **–IBS Unclassified (IBS-U)** | IBS in which bowel habits cannot be accurately categorized into one of the three classifications listed above. |
| **C2. Functional Constipation** | Defecation is usually difficult, infrequent, or incomplete. Abdominal pain or bloating may be present but do not predominate (as they do with IBS-C). Patients meeting criteria for IBS-C should be excluded. **http://bit.ly/2HCBiV1** **https://romedross.video/11_15_19IBSCD** |
| **C3. Functional Diarrhea** | Loose or watery stools, without predominant abdominal pain or bothersome bloating, occurring 25% of the time or more. Patients meeting criteria for IBS-D should be excluded. **https://romedross.video/2GJIEnt** |
| **C4. Functional Abdominal Bloating/Distension** | Recurrent bloating and/or distension of the abdomen that occurs on average at least 1 day a week and predominates over other symptoms. Patients with other bowel disorders, as listed above, should be excluded. **http://bit.ly/2NHQH5i** |
| **C5. Unspecified Functional Bowel Disorder** | Bowel symptoms, including abdominal pain or change in bowel habits that do not have an organic cause and do not meet criteria for IBS or functional constipation, diarrhea, or abdominal bloating/distention disorders. |
| **C6. Opioid-Induced Constipation** | New or worsening symptoms of constipation when initiating, changing, or increasing opioid therapy. **http://bit.ly/2Pm9wLV** |

| D. Centrally Mediated Disorders of Gastrointestinal Pain[19] | |
|---|---|
| **Functional Disorder** | **Functional definition and links to more information** |
| **D1. Centrally Mediated Abdominal Pain Syndrome (CAPS)** | Continuous, nearly continuous, or frequently recurrent abdominal pain that is often severe and not or rarely related to changes in gut function such as eating or defecation. The pain is not feigned nor related to another gastrointestinal disorder. **https://romedross.video/2ZbDTcW** |
| **D2. Narcotic Bowel Syndrome (NBS) / Opioid-Induced GI Hyperalgesia** | Development of (or increases in) abdominal pain associated with continuous or increasing dosages of opioids. The pain is not explained by other medical diagnoses. When opioid use ends, improvement or resolution will occur. **http://bit.ly/2Pm9wLV** |

| E. Gallbladder and Sphincter of Oddi (SO) Disorders[20] | |
|---|---|
| **Functional Disorder** | **Functional definition and links to more information** |
| **E1. Biliary Pain** | Pain that is episodic and located in the epigastrium (upper central region of the abdomen) and/or right upper quadrant that lasts 30 minutes or longer and is severe enough to interrupt daily activities or lead to an emergency room visit. **https://romedross.video/2KcceGh** |
| **-E1a. Functional Gall-bladder Disorder** | Biliary pain (see E1) in the absence of gallstones or other structural pathology. **https://romedross.video/2KcceGh** |
| **-E1b. Functional Biliary Sphincter of Oddi (SO) Disorder** | Biliary pain (see E1) in the absence of bile duct stones or other structural abnormalities that is associated with abnormal liver enzymes or a dilated bile duct (but not both). Often, the gallbladder has been surgically removed. **https://romedross.video/2KcceGh** |
| **E2. Functional Pancreatic SO Disorder** | Biliary pain (see E1) associated with episodes of pancreatitis (inflammation of the pancreas associated with elevated pancreatic enzymes). Patients with unexplained attacks of pancreatitis are often found to have elevated pancreatic sphincter pressure. |

| F. Anorectal Disorders[21] | |
|---|---|
| **Functional Disorder** | **Functional definition and links to more information** |
| **F1. Fecal Incontinence** | Recurrent uncontrolled passage of fecal material for at least 3 months. |
| **F2. Functional Anorectal Pain** | Three types of functional anorectal pain disorders have been described and are explained below (see F2a, F2b, F2c). They are primarily distinguished by the duration of pain and the presence or absence of anorectal tenderness but overlap significantly. **https://romedross.video/QA1_24_20PFD** **https://romedross.video/Q_A_RectalPainExam** |
| **-F2a. Levator Ani Syndrome** | Pain that is often described as a vague, dull ache, or a sensation of pressure high in the rectum lasting 30 minutes or longer. It is often worse when sitting than when standing or lying down. Physical examination reveals tenderness when the doctor presses on the pelvic floor (posterior traction of the levator) muscle. Other structural disorders of the pelvic floor must be excluded. **https://romedross.video/34cjdXS** |
| **-F2b. Unspecified Functional Anorectal Pain** | Same symptoms as Levator Ani Syndrome, but upon rectal exam, there is no tenderness when the doctor presses on the levator muscle. |
| **-F2c. Proctalgia Fugax** | Recurrent episodes of pain in the rectal area, lasting for a few seconds to several minutes (up to 30 minutes) and then disappearing completely. It has been described as cramping, gnawing, aching, or stabbing, and may range from uncomfortable to unbearable. An attack may interrupt normal activities, and symptoms may awaken the patient from sleep. |
| **F3. Functional Defecation Disorders (FDD)** | Also called pelvic floor dyssynergia. Frequent excessive straining, feeling of incomplete evacuation with defecation, and at times digital facilitation of bowel movements. The pelvic floor muscles contract with defecation, rather than relaxing, as they should, or there is not enough pressure (propulsive force) to defecate (see F3a and F3b). **http://bit.ly/2C3VCMO** |
| **-F3a. Inadequate Defecatory Propulsion** | Inadequate propulsive force to defecate properly. **http://bit.ly/2HCBiV1** |
| **-F3b. Dyssynergic Defecation** | Inappropriate or paradoxical contraction of the pelvic floor with failure to relax the levator muscle (puborectalis), associated with straining and difficulty with evacuating. **http://bit.ly/2HCBiV1** |

| G. Childhood Functional GI Disorders: Neonate/Toddler (Age 0–4)[22] | |
|---|---|
| **Functional Disorder** | **Functional definition** |
| **G1. Infant Regurgitation** | The involuntary return of swallowed food or secretions into or out of the esophagus, mouth, or nose. It differs from vomiting, which involves a reflex in which gastric contents are forcefully expelled. |
| **G2. Rumination Syndrome** | Habitual regurgitation of stomach contents into the mouth for self-stimulation caused by repetitive contractions of the abdominal muscles. |
| **G3. Cyclic Vomiting Syndrome (CVS)** | Stereotypical and repeated episodes of vomiting without retching that last from hours to days, with intervening periods of return to baseline normal health. Typically, vomiting episodes are separated by weeks or months. |
| **G4. Infant Colic** | Behavioral syndrome of early infancy (less than 5 months of age) involving recurrent or prolonged periods of crying, fussing, irritability, and hard-to-soothe behavior. More likely to occur in the afternoon or evening. |
| **G5. Functional Diarrhea** | Daily and recurrent painless passage of four or more large, un-formed stools for 4 or more weeks, beginning in infancy or pre-school years. No evidence of failure to thrive. |
| **G6. Infant Dyschezia** | Straining for at least 10 minutes, with crying, before the successful or unsuccessful passage of soft stools. The child may turn red or purple in the face with each effort to defecate. Symptoms usually persist for 10–20 minutes. Stools pass several times a day. |
| **G7. Functional Constipation** | Infrequent (two or fewer per week) or painful defecation in infants and toddlers associated with excessive stool retention and/or hard or large-diameter stools; in older children, it may be related to fecal incontinence and withholding behavior. |

| H. Childhood Functional GI Disorders: Child/Adolescent (Age 5 and older)[23] | |
|---|---|
| **Functional Disorder** | **Functional definition and link to more information** |
| **H1. Functional Nausea and Vomiting Disorders** | Nausea is an unpleasant feeling, usually in the epigastrium or throat, associated with a sense of needing to vomit. Vomiting is the forceful expulsion of upper gastrointestinal contents following the contraction of gut and the thoracic and abdominal muscles. It is different from regurgitation or rumination, in which the movement of gastric contents into the mouth is effortless. See H1a and H1b, below, for definitions of the sub-classifications. **http://bit.ly/2wW5hiD** |
| **-H1a. Cyclic Vomiting Syndrome (CVS)** | Stereotypical and repeated episodes of intense vomiting, separated by weeks or months, and with a return to baseline health between episodes. |
| **-H1b. Functional Nausea and Functional Vomiting** | These disorders are sub-classified and described below (see H1b1 and H1b2). |
| **-H1b1. Functional Nausea** | Bothersome nausea is the predominant symptom, occurring at least twice a week, and generally not related to meals. |
| **-H1b2. Functional Vomiting** | On average, one or more episodes of vomiting per week that are not self-induced or related to an eating disorder or rumination. |
| **-H1c. Rumination Syndrome** | Repeated regurgitation into the mouth of recently eaten food, with subsequent re-swallowing or expulsion. The symptom begins soon after ingestion of a meal, is not associated with retching, and does not occur during sleep. |
| **-H1d. Aerophagia** | Excessive swallowing of air that causes abdominal distension, which becomes progressively worse during the day. Air swallowing may be visible, is often audible, and results in excessive belching or flatus. |
| **H2. Functional Abdominal Pain Disorders** | Disorders in which pain is the main symptom. These are sub-classified and defined below (see H2a, H2a1, H2a2, H2b, H2c, and H2d). |
| **-H2a. Functional Dyspepsia** | Upper gastrointestinal discomfort that may include a combination of unpleasant features, including a sensation of fullness after eating, early satiety, or upper abdominal pain or burning. The symptoms can cause significant impairment in quality of life. |
| **-H2a1. Postprandial Distress Syndrome** | Bothersome fullness soon after a meal or early satiety that prevents finishing a regular-sized meal. May include upper abdominal bloating, nausea, or excessive belching. |

*continues*

| H. Childhood Functional GI Disorders: Child/Adolescent (Age 5 and older)[23] | |
|---|---|
| **Functional Disorder** | **Functional definition and link to more information** |
| **-H2a2. Epigastric Pain Syndrome** | Bothersome pain or burning localized to the epigastrium (severe enough to interfere with normal activities). Pain is not generalized or localized to other abdominal or chest regions and is not relieved by defecation or passage of flatus. |
| **-H2b. Irritable Bowel Syndrome (IBS)** | Abdominal discomfort or pain associated with defecation or disordered defecation, and a change in the frequency and form (appearance) of the stool. |
| **-H2c. Abdominal Migraine** | Short but intense and paroxysmal episodes of abdominal pain lasting 1 hour or more, commonly separated by weeks to months, and associated with incapacitating symptoms that interfere with activities. Symptoms are often associated with loss of appetite, nausea and vomiting, headache, sensitivity to light, and pale skin. |
| **-H2d. Functional Abdominal Pain—NOS** | Episodic or continuous abdominal pain not related to eating or defecation at least four times a month that do not meet the criteria for IBS, functional dyspepsia, or abdominal migraine. |
| **H3. Functional Defecation Disorders** | These disorders relate to symptoms associated with the passage of stool. They are sub-classified and described below (see H3a and H3b). |
| **-H3a. Functional Constipation** | Infrequent bowel movements (two or fewer per week), associated with painful passage of hard stools, the passage of a large-diameter stool, or fecal incontinence. Involuntary leakage of feces may occur several times a day if a rectal impaction is present. |
| **-H3b. Nonretentive Fecal Incontinence** | Repeated passage of stool in a place inappropriate for the social context that is not associated with fecal retention. |

Now that we have given you a brief definition and description of all the DGBI classified by Rome IV, we want to provide you with more information on these disorders. For each diagnosis, we will provide a general overview and definition, the pathophysiology (the reasons why the symptoms occur), the clinical features, the diagnostic evaluation (including the Rome IV criteria), and the treatment. The Rome IV book contains a comprehensive discussion of all these diagnoses.[24] **It is important to remember that the diagnosis of DGBI always requires that (1) the doctor fulfill the Rome IV diagnostic criteria (see Appendix A), (2) the doctor excludes structural abnormalities and other causes that might explain the symptoms, and (3) the Rome IV criteria are fulfilled for at least 3 months, and the symptoms began at least 6 months before diagnosis.**

## A. Esophageal Disorders[16]

Esophageal symptoms are common and easy to locate under the sternum or breastbone. The symptoms may include difficulty swallowing, called dysphagia (feels like food is getting stuck as it goes down), pain, regurgitation of liquid or food, and heartburn. These symptoms may have structural causes like Gastroesophageal Reflux Disease (GERD), esophageal strictures or blockages, or motility problems. However, functional esophageal disorders consist of symptoms that patients locate in the chest and that cannot be explained by any structural abnormalities in the esophagus or other cardiac or pulmonary disease. Upper endoscopy should be normal, and with older patients, heart disease must be excluded.

Underlying reasons for the symptoms of the functional esophageal disorders may include hypersensitivity of the esophagus, alterations in the way the brain processes nerve impulses coming from the gut, altered motor function (motility), and altered activity in the part of the nervous system that regulates esophageal functioning.

### A1. Functional Chest Pain

Have you ever seen someone with chest pain believe they have a heart attack, but instead, get diagnosed with "esophageal spasm"? That's because Functional Chest Pain is recurring, unexplained pain or discomfort behind the sternum. However, Functional Chest Pain is far more common than coronary disease in young and middle-aged adults who are otherwise healthy; it is due to increased sensitivity of the nerves in the esophagus (visceral hypersensitivity) or abnormal motility. Certainly, cardiac causes must be ruled out, especially in older patients or those at high risk, because the sensation may be similar. Usually, Gastroesophageal Reflux Disease (GERD), where increased acid enters the esophagus and causes inflammation or ulcers, needs to be excluded. The doctor must also eliminate esophageal or stomach blockage (such as a stricture or tumor) or an esophageal motility disorder (e.g., diffuse esophageal spasm). Some patients experience these as similar to angina, and this is often called Non-Cardiac Chest Pain (NCCP).

Esophageal chest pain often is associated with psychological distress, such as anxiety and depression, and sleep difficulties are more common than in healthy individuals. Heightened pain perception usually exists and is due to the visceral hypersensitivity of the esophagus. Visceral hypersensitivity occurs with normal stretching of the esophagus (such as when one swallows), with acid reflux, or even in a resting state without any provocation.

***Pathophysiology.*** Studies consistently show altered pain perception and visceral hypersensitivity to be the hallmark of Functional Chest Pain. This can begin with injury to the esophageal tissue, or with inflammation, or for no apparent reason at all. Notably, esophageal hypersensitivity can remain long after the original cause has been resolved. It may be a result of enhanced processing at the level of the brain and spinal cord (central hypersensitivity; see D. Centrally Mediated Disorders of GI Pain).

***Clinical Evaluation.***

> **Rome IV Criteria for Functional Chest Pain (A1)**
>
> Must include all of the following:
>
> 1. Retrosternal chest pain or discomfort; cardiac causes should be ruled out
> 2. Absence of associated esophageal symptoms, such as heartburn and dysphagia
> 3. Absence of evidence that gastroesophageal reflux or eosinophilic esophagitis (EoE) are the cause of the symptom
> 4. Absence of major esophageal motor disorders (achalasia/esophagogastric junction (EGJ) outflow obstruction, diffuse esophageal spasm, jackhammer esophagus, absent peristalsis)

Clinical evaluation includes meeting Rome IV criteria and excluding other diagnoses such as GERD, esophageal motility disorders, or structural findings such as an esophageal stricture or obstruction. Upper endoscopy is usually needed to eliminate these disorders, and in older patients, coronary disease needs to be excluded.

***Treatment.*** No one treatment for Functional Chest Pain is useful for everyone. Management of the disorder involves medications that reduce pain, coupled with psychotherapy, cognitive behavioral therapy, biofeedback, or hypnotherapy. A range of neuromodulators (i.e., antidepressants) have pain-relieving properties that are separate from their effect on mood, and they can ease the pain even when there is no mood disorder. Serotonin reuptake inhibitors such as Prozac (fluoxetine) or Celexa (citalopram), and tricyclic antidepressants (TCAs) such as Elavil (amitriptyline) have been studied and show benefits.[25]

Psychological treatments, including cognitive-behavioral therapy (CBT) or hypnosis, show overall benefit. Patients who appreciate the fact that the esophagus is the source of their pain (as opposed to a coronary reason, for example) are less likely to be disabled by their symptoms, just by having that knowledge.

## A2. Functional Heartburn

Functional Heartburn describes a burning discomfort or pain behind the sternum when there is no injury to the lining of the esophagus and no increase in acid reflux—nor is there any correlation between these symptoms and the presence of acid reflux as measured by pH testing. When increased amounts of acid are present and result in damage to the esophagus, the diagnosis is Gastroesophageal Reflux Disease (GERD). Almost 70% of patients with heartburn symptoms have no evidence of esophageal injury. When there is an increased amount of acid reflux with no injury to the esophagus, the diagnosis is Non-Erosive Reflux Disease (NERD). However, when there is heartburn, no increased acid reflux, and no relationship between heartburn and reflux, the diagnosis is Functional Heartburn. In other words, the diagnosis of Functional Heartburn occurs after excluding GERD and NERD. Since the sensation of heartburn is the same for all these disorders, the diagnosis of these disorders usually requires endoscopic and physiological pH testing (the measurement of acid going from the stomach to the esophagus).

***Pathophysiology.*** The mechanism of symptom generation in Functional Heartburn is unclear, but the prevailing view is that altered esophageal visceral hypersensitivity is a significant factor. Other possible reasons include central hypersensitivity in the parts of the brain that control pain and can be activated by psychological distress, much like that seen with other painful DGBI. Patients with Functional Heartburn demonstrate higher levels of anxiety than do patients with GERD, and Functional Heartburn frequently co-exists in people with other DGBI, such as Functional Dyspepsia, Functional Chest Pain, and Irritable Bowel Syndrome (to be discussed later). Since the heartburn is not due to increased acid reflux, one hypothesis relates to increased permeability of the mucous lining (akin to "leaky gut" often described to occur in the bowel in IBS). This may allow harmful, sensitizing substances to access the deeper layers of the esophagus, where they may induce an inflammatory response that sensitizes these nerves. Also, abnormal central processing of signals from the esophagus can support the generation of symptoms without an event that triggers reflux.

***Clinical Evaluation.***

**Rome IV Criteria for Functional Heartburn (A2)**

Must include all of the following:

1. Burning retrosternal discomfort or pain
2. No symptom relief despite optimal antisecretory therapy
3. Absence of evidence that gastroesophageal reflux (abnormal acid exposure and symptom reflux association) or EoE is the cause of symptoms
4. Absence of major esophageal motor disorders (achalasia/EGJ outflow obstruction, diffuse esophageal spasm, jackhammer esophagus, absent peristalsis)

Similar to the evaluation of Functional Chest Pain, the patient must meet Rome IV criteria; then an upper endoscopy must exclude structural esophageal disorders and determine if esophageal damage (e.g., ulcers, erosions, or strictures) have occurred from GERD. A pH study may be done by placing a tube through the nose or endoscopically into the stomach to measure acidity and determine how heartburn symptoms and acid reflux correlate. When the results of these tests are negative, the diagnosis is Functional Heartburn.

***Treatment.*** Although commonly used, patients with Functional Heartburn do not respond well to medications designed to decrease acid secretion, such as antacids, H2 blockers (e.g., Pepcid, Zantac), or protein pump inhibitors (e.g., Prilosec or Nexium). Even though increased acid does not cause the pain, doctors commonly prescribe them because they are safe, and the symptoms may spontaneously resolve over time. Treatment is based primarily on observing how well or poorly a remedy works. What is essential is that the doctor educate the patient on the nature of the disorders (which is often therapeutic by itself) and avoid unneeded endoscopy and other diagnostic studies after initially excluding other diseases. Pain modulators like low-dose tricyclic antidepressants such as Elavil (amitriptyline), and selective serotonin reuptake inhibitors (SSRIs) such as Celexa (citalopram) and Prozac (fluoxetine), may be tried and have empiric value. When implemented in conjunction with the psychological interventions described above for Functional Chest Pain, these measures can be helpful for patients with more severe symptoms.

## A3. Reflux Hypersensitivity

This new Rome IV diagnosis is defined by heartburn or chest pain when there is no evidence of acid damage (seen on endoscopy) or abnormal acid reflux into the esophagus from the stomach (based on measuring acid reflux through pH testing). In these patients, even normal degrees of acid reflux trigger symptoms; in other words, they are hypersensitive to usual degrees of acid. Some patients meeting this diagnosis may respond to anti-reflux measures. Still, the underlying cause is more consistent with the hypersensitivity of the esophagus (i.e., acid-sensitive nerve receptors in the esophagus fire more frequently in response to normal acid stimuli). Furthermore, an overlap may exist between true GERD, where there is acid damage and reflux hypersensitivity.

***Pathophysiology.*** Reflux Hypersensitivity symptoms are much like Functional Chest Pain and Functional Heartburn, with the caveat that normal degrees of acid reflux events (based on pH testing) trigger symptoms. Also, how the brain experiences these signals (central hypersensitivity) can be worsened by stress and altered emotional states like anxiety, and lead to hypersensitivity of the esophagus and symptoms.

***Clinical Evaluation.***

**Rome IV Criteria for Reflux Hypersensitivity (A3)**

Must include all of the following:

1. Retrosternal symptoms including heartburn and chest pain
2. Normal endoscopy and absence of evidence that EoE is the cause for symptoms
3. Absence of major esophageal motor disorders (achalasia/EGJ outflow obstruction, diffuse esophageal spasm, jackhammer esophagus, absent peristalsis)
4. Evidence of triggering of symptoms by reflux events despite normal acid exposure on pH or pH-impedance monitoring (response to antisecretory therapy does not exclude the diagnosis)

The clinical presentation of patients with Reflux Hypersensitivity is the same as those with Functional Heartburn and NERD. Upper endoscopy is done to rule out other conditions, and esophageal motility testing may be done to rule out major motility disorders such as esophageal spasm. Determining sensitivity to normal degrees of acid reflux by pH testing is the hallmark for diagnosis. Even though the amount of acid entering the esophagus is normal (unlike NERD or GERD), the presence of acid produces heartburn; this is called an increased symptom association. The doctor may also initiate a diagnostic trial by prescribing a proton pump inhibitor (PPI) such as Nexium (esomeprazole) or Prilosec (omeprazole).

***Treatment.*** As in the management of Functional Heartburn, the doctor must educate and provide reassurance. Patients should be counseled that no other ominous diagnosis exists. As noted, patients with Reflux Hypersensitivity may respond better to antisecretory therapy than do individuals with Functional Heartburn or other functional esophageal disorders. The mainstay of treatment for Esophageal Hypersensitivity, when PPIs don't work, are pain neuromodulators, including TCAs such as Elavil (amitriptyline), SSRIs such as Celexa (citalopram), serotonin noradrenergic reuptake inhibitors such as Cymbalta (duloxetine), and gabapentenoids such as Neurontin (gabapentin). Some doctors have done anti-reflux surgery, but this is controversial.

## A4. Globus

Have you ever stopped yourself from crying in a sad movie or at a wedding and felt like you had "a lump in your throat"? This sensation is similar to Globus: a persistent or intermittent *non-painful* sensation of a lump or foreign body in the throat. The symptom occurs in the midline in the lower throat above the sternal notch. It is episodic, not related to difficulty swallowing (Dysphagia), and often improves with eating and drinking. Diagnosis of Globus requires the absence of structural abnormalities in the mucous lining or major motor disorders.

***Pathophysiology.*** Globus sensation may feel like a blockage or like acid reflux, or it may be related to a motility disorder. When these disorders are excluded, Globus is related to abnormal visceral hypersensitivity and the heightened central processing of esophageal stimuli seen with other functional esophageal disorders. Mild distension of the esophagus with a balloon can reproduce the sensation of Globus, suggesting esophageal hypersensitivity. Although Globus can occur in patients having GERD, it does not respond well to anti-reflux therapy. When Globus sensation is frequent, I find it helpful to explore emotional factors like significant loss or grief, as this symptom may be a physiological expression of suppressed emotion.

***Clinical Evaluation.***

**Rome IV Criteria for Globus (A4)**

Must include all of the following:

1. Persistent or intermittent, non-painful sensation of a lump or foreign body in the throat with no structural lesion identified on physical examination, laryngoscopy, or endoscopy
   a. Occurrence of the sensation between meals
   b. Absence of dysphagia or odynophagia
   c. Absence of a gastric inlet patch in the proximal esophagus
2. Absence of evidence that gastroesophageal reflux or EoE is the cause of the symptom
3. Absence of major esophageal motor disorders (achalasia/EGJ outflow obstruction, diffuse esophageal spasm, jackhammer esophagus, absent peristalsis)

As with other functional esophageal disorders, the diagnosis of Globus is made primarily by eliciting a clinical history that fits the Rome IV criteria and excluding other identifiable causes, such as a structural lesion, GERD, or a major motor disorder. Typically, there is no dysphagia (trouble swallowing) or painful swallowing (odynophagia). The doctor should do a physical examination of the neck and throat, and at times the patient may need to be referred to an ear, nose, and throat specialist to have a laryngoscopic examination of the pharynx. Once structural or inflammatory causes have been excluded, the doctor can do a diagnostic trial using a PPI for 4–8 weeks. If the patient responds well, treatment continues with this medication. If the patient does not respond, the doctor may do an upper endoscopy to assess for structural causes possibly overlooked. Esophageal motor testing (manometry) may be helpful to rule out a motility disorder but is usually normal. When patients do not respond to PPI and have no identifiable cause in the oropharynx and esophagus, Globus is the diagnosis.

***Treatment.*** Since this is a benign condition, symptoms, explanation, and reassurance are the mainstays of therapy for Globus. If emotional contributing factors exist, referral to a mental health provider for further evaluation and treatment may be of value. In this case, I would also prescribe a central neuromodulator to reduce the influence of stress or symptoms associated with anxiety or depression, thereby reducing the frequency or severity of the symptoms.

## A5. Functional Dysphagia

If you had Dysphagia when you were young, your parent might have said, "*Eat slowly and chew your food*"! People may experience Dysphagia when they swallow a large piece of food too quickly. This diagnosis is characterized by a feeling of a blockage in the esophagus as the food is going down. Narrowing of the esophagus by a stricture or a motility disorder may also cause Dysphagia. Diagnosis, therefore, requires exclusion of any structural causes of Dysphagia in the esophagus, or evidence for GERD or other major motor disorder.

***Pathophysiology.*** The relationship between food getting stuck and the sensation of Dysphagia is not perfect. The way food goes down the esophagus can depend on its consistency and dryness; it can take several swallows to clear dry food, even in otherwise healthy individuals. The sensation of dysphagia may also be caused by posture, as it's more difficult to eat when lying down than sitting up. While these symptoms are often diagnosed as "spasm" or abnormal contractions, evidence for esophageal motility abnormalities causing spasm is difficult to confirm. Certain motility disorders, like achalasia or diffuse esophageal spasm, are associated with the esophagus over-contracting or not contracting enough, so we need to exclude these motility disorders. Rather than being a motility problem, Functional Dysphagia appears to result from esophageal hypersensitivity. The feeling of food sticking can be induced by distending a balloon or acidifying the esophagus.

***Clinical Evaluation.***

**Rome IV Criteria for Functional Dysphagia (A5)**

Must include all of the following:

1. Sense of solid and/or liquid foods sticking, lodging, or passing abnormally through the esophagus
2. Absence of evidence that esophageal mucosal or structural abnormality is the cause of the symptom
3. Absence of evidence that gastroesophageal reflux or EoE is the cause of the symptom
4. Absence of major esophageal motor disorders (achalasia/EGJ outflow obstruction, diffuse esophageal spasm, jackhammer esophagus, absent peristalsis)

The doctor should take a careful history to exclude structural causes for dysphagia or other conditions mimicking or contributing to dysphagia (i.e., Globus, diseases causing dry mouth, or infectious causes of painful swallowing like odynophagia).

GERD and eosinophilic esophagitis (EOE) may produce dysphagia, and I typically treat with PPI therapy and do an upper endoscopy combined with biopsy. Barium contrast studies, especially using a tablet, cookie, or marshmallow (to replicate food going through the esophagus), can evaluate for subtle strictures and certain types of hiatal hernias that are often overlooked on endoscopy. If no structural lesions are found, esophageal manometry is done to exclude major motor disorders like achalasia or diffuse esophageal spasm.

***Treatment.*** Functional Dysphagia may get better over time, and aggressive management approaches may not be necessary. Reassurance and simple measures such as eating in the upright position, avoiding food items that trigger it, careful chewing of food, and chasing food with liquids may suffice in mild cases. A short trial of PPI may be useful because Dysphagia can be part of the reflux spectrum. Central neuromodulators, such as TCAs, can be tried. The use of an esophageal dilator or bougie showed to benefit 68–85% of patients who have intermittent food dysphagia without an identifiable source.

## B. Gastroduodenal Disorders[17]

Gastroduodenal disorders involve symptoms that are presumed to arise in the stomach and the duodenum (the first part of the small intestine, immediately beneath the stomach). Occasional symptoms are often called "indigestion" or "upset stomach." Interestingly, the Italian term "agida" is the word for both discomforts of the upper gut and stress. The most common of these disorders is Functional Dyspepsia (FD), an over-arching term that is sub-classified into different syndromes according to the type of symptoms experienced as described below.

### B1. Functional Dyspepsia (FD)

How does it feel when you eat too large a meal at Thanksgiving? That describes the cardinal symptoms associated with Functional Dyspepsia. It is a common, chronic disorder characterized by one or more of the following: (1) unpleasant sensation of prolonged persistence of food in the stomach after a meal ("postprandial fullness"); (2) unpleasant feeling that the stomach is over-filled soon after starting to eat, out of proportion to the actual size of the meal, and such that one can't finish the meal ("early satiety"); (3) intense, unpleasant pain in the upper abdomen ("epigastric pain"); or (4) unpleasant sensation of burning or heat in the upper abdomen ("epigastric burning"). When these symptoms remain unexplained by routine clinical evaluation, including upper endoscopy, the diagnosis is Functional Dyspepsia (FD). FD is sub-classified into two sub-syndromes (**https://romedross.video/36uTGaA**):

**B1a. Postprandial Distress Syndrome (PDS)** – occurs when symptoms are meal-induced. Eating a meal leads to feeling full after a meal (postprandial fullness) and/or early satiety at least 3 days a week. It may include upper abdominal (epigastric) pain after eating, as well as bloating, belching, and nausea.

**B1b. Epigastric Pain Syndrome (EPS)** – occurs when epigastric pain or burning may occur during fasting or after meals. Symptoms of EPS must occur at least 1 day a week to fit this classification.

***Pathophysiology.*** The pathophysiology of FD is complex and may have multiple causes. Several possibilities include delayed gastric emptying, impaired gastric accommodation, and gastric hypersensitivity. There is, however, evidence that acute infection can trigger the symptoms of FD (this is post-infection dyspepsia). PDS seems to occur when the stomach fails to relax and expand properly to accommodate food after eating; increased tension of the stomach wall produces symptoms of bloating and early satiety. EPS, on the other hand, may relate more to visceral hypersensitivity.

Physiological abnormalities associated with these diagnoses include abnormal gastric and duodenal motility, impaired mucosal integrity (i.e., increased permeability – "leaky gut"), low-grade immune abnormalities, and inflammation. There are also alterations of the brain-gut axis that lead to anxiety and depression.

The emptying of food from the stomach may be slightly delayed but does not usually relate to the symptoms of Functional Dyspepsia.

Eating a meal stretches the stomach and stimulates the vagus nerve, causing a vasovagal reflex where the nerve signals go from the stomach to the brain and then back to the stomach, causing it to relax (gastric accommodation). Patients with FD, especially PDS, have impairment of this reflex, thereby reducing gastric relaxation after a meal, and this is associated with early satiety. Hypersensitivity to mechanical stimulation of the stomach and upper small bowel is also frequent in FD patients. *H. pylori* infection can also cause FD symptoms, and treating this infection may improve the symptoms in a small percentage of patients. Some patients with FD have increased duodenal inflammatory cells, called eosinophils. Duodenal eosinophilia, when present, is associated with early satiety. Other factors implicating the development of symptoms include infection, stress, duodenal acid exposure, smoking, and food allergies, all of which can lead to inflammation and increased permeability of the duodenal mucosal lining.

*Clinical Evaluation.*

**Rome IV Criteria for Functional Dyspepsia (B1)**

Must include:

1. One or more of the following:
   a. Bothersome postprandial fullness
   b. Bothersome early satiation
   c. Bothersome epigastric pain
   d. Bothersome epigastric burning

AND

2. No evidence of structural disease (including at upper endoscopy) that is likely to explain the symptoms. Must fulfill criteria for B1a PDS and/or B1b EPS.

---

**B1a. Postprandial Distress Syndrome (PDS)**

Must include one or both of the following at least 3 days per week:

1. Bothersome postprandial fullness (i.e., severe enough to impact on usual activities)
2. Bothersome early satiation (i.e., severe enough to prevent finishing a regular-size meal)

No evidence of organic, systemic, or metabolic disease that is likely to explain the symptoms on routine investigations (including at upper endoscopy)

*Supportive criteria:*

1. Postprandial epigastric pain or burning, epigastric bloating, excessive belching, and nausea can also be present
2. Vomiting warrants consideration of another disorder
3. Heartburn is not a dyspeptic symptom but may often co-exist
4. Symptoms that are relieved by evacuation of feces or gas should generally not be considered as part of dyspepsia
5. Other individual digestive symptoms or groups of symptoms, e.g., from gastroesophageal reflux disease and irritable bowel syndrome may co-exist with PDS

---

**B1b. Epigastric Pain Syndrome (EPS)**

Must include at least one of the following symptoms at least 1 day a week:

1. Bothersome epigastric pain (i.e., severe enough to impact on usual activities)

AND/OR

2. Bothersome epigastric burning (i.e., severe enough to impact on usual activities)

No evidence of organic, systemic, or metabolic disease that is likely to explain the symptoms on routine investigations (including at upper endoscopy)

*Supportive criteria:*

1. Pain may be induced by ingestion of a meal, relieved by ingestion of a meal, or may occur while fasting
2. Postprandial epigastric bloating, belching, and nausea can also be present
3. Persistent vomiting likely suggests another disorder
4. Heartburn is not a dyspeptic symptom but may often co-exist
5. The pain does not fulfill biliary pain criteria
6. Symptoms that are relieved by evacuation of feces or gas generally should not be considered as part of dyspepsia
7. Other digestive symptoms (such as from gastroesophageal reflux disease and the irritable bowel syndrome) may co-exist with EPS

When the symptoms fulfill Rome IV criteria, the next step would be for the doctor to check for "alarm" signals that might prompt further diagnostic evaluation. Alarm signals include blood in the stool, weight loss, or an abnormal physical examination (e.g., abdominal mass, localized tenderness). At this point, the patient has un-investigated dyspepsia. However, because ulcers, tumors, and strictures of the stomach and duodenum may cause FD symptoms, an upper endoscopy is often needed to exclude these diagnoses. Furthermore, *H. pylori*, a bacterial infection in the stomach, can also produce dyspeptic symptoms, so the doctor may order an endoscopic biopsy or breath-study testing. If the *H. pylori* testing is positive, the symptoms may improve by treating the infection with antibiotics. If endoscopy is negative, then FD is the diagnosis. At this point, sub-classifying the symptoms may be helpful. As noted, patients with meal-related early satiety or fullness are usually diagnosed as PDS, while those without meal-related symptoms of burning or pain have EPS; however, these two categories often co-exist.

FD may be confused with gastroparesis, which is a motility disorder, not a DGBI. Gastroparesis is diagnosed by showing markedly delayed gastric emptying on a gastric emptying radionuclide study. Severe gastroparesis produces vomiting, loss of appetite, and weight loss. However, mild gastroparesis (with mildly delayed gastric emptying) may produce no symptoms at all. Diagnosing between FD and gastroparesis is often confusing. Most of the time, patients carrying a diagnosis of gastroparesis may come to see me. However, there is usually mildly delayed gastric emptying, and the symptoms are due to FD.

***Treatment.*** Because a large proportion of otherwise healthy individuals have dyspepsia and because endoscopy is expensive, the doctor may consider first treating un-investigated dyspepsia before doing an upper endoscopy. Management of un-investigated dyspepsia is determined by taking a careful history and treating possibly overlapping GERD, and *H. pylori*, especially in areas where *H. pylori* infection is common ("test and treat"). However, if alarm features are present, upper endoscopy should be performed. Treatment of Functional Dyspepsia involves reassurance from the provider, as well as education, lifestyle, and dietary recommendations (i.e., more frequent, smaller meals with less fat content). Patients are also often advised to avoid nonsteroidal anti-inflammatory drugs, coffee, alcohol, and smoking—all of which seem sensible, even though its scientific value has not been established.

If FD is diagnosed and endoscopy is negative, patients should be divided into PDS and/or EPS and treated accordingly, because each sub-category may have different treatments.

Treatment relates primarily to medications and psychological therapies. Since the PDS subtype appears to refer to the failure of the stomach to relax when receiving food, Buspar (buspirone), a gastric-relaxing agent, may be tried. Outside the USA, medications such as Itopride, a promotility agent, and Acotiamide, a gastric, fundus-relaxing agent, have been shown to improve dyspeptic symptoms.

In EPS, visceral hypersensitivity may help to explain the pain. Doctors may first prescribe an H2 acid blocker such as Pepcid (famotidine) or Tagamet (cimetidine), or a proton-pump inhibitor such as Prilosec (omeprazole) or Nexium (esomeprazole). This is based on the assumption that acid reduction may help. Neuromodulators (antidepressants), particularly the tricyclic class (TCAs), can be useful in patients with FD. Certain promotility drugs, especially those with a combined antiemetic action (such as metoclopramide) may also be considered. Psychological therapies, such as cognitive-behavioral treatment, have also shown benefit, especially when the associated symptoms of anxiety and depression or health worry are present.

## B2. Belching Disorders

Everyone belches. It is a normal physiological function—an audible escape of air from the esophagus or the stomach into the pharynx—and it is commonly glorified by children and adolescents showing off. Because belching is so frequent, it is considered a medical disorder only when the belching is excessive and troublesome to the patient or others. Depending on the origin of the refluxed gas, belching has two subtypes:

**B2a. Excessive Supragastric Belching (from the esophagus)**

**B2b. Excessive Gastric Belching (from the stomach)**

***Pathophysiology.*** When air is swallowed, it is transported to the stomach along with the rest of the food or liquid and accumulates in the upper part of the stomach. A venting system protects the stomach against extreme stretching, and the lower esophageal sphincter (LES) acts as a barrier to air or food going from the stomach into the esophagus. When the stomach is distended or stretched by gas, the LES relaxes, leading the gas to escape into the esophagus. Then the upper esophageal sphincter (UES) relaxes, and the air escapes, causing the belch.

In most patients, supragastric belches occur only in the esophagus. The diaphragm moves down, as it does when you breathe deeply. This leads to a lowering of pressure in the thoracic (chest) cavity, which traps the air in the esophagus, and it is then released. In contrast, gastric belches occur when air escapes from the stomach because intrathoracic pressure is elevated when the LES is relaxed. UES relaxation occurs in both supragastric and gastric belches. Supragastric belching stops during speaking, distraction, and sleeping. It is often associated with stressful events and anxiety states and can impair health-related quality of life. Excessive belching can occur with anxiety, obsessive-compulsive disorder, and bulimia nervosa.

***Clinical Evaluation.***

**Rome IV Criteria for Belching Disorders (B2)**

Must include all of the following:

Bothersome (i.e., severe enough to impact on usual activities) belching from the esophagus or stomach more than 3 days a week

**B2a: Excessive supragastric belching (from esophagus)**

**B2b: Excessive gastric belching (from stomach)**

*Supportive criteria:*

1. Supragastric belching is supported by observing frequent, repetitive belching
2. Gastric belching has no established clinical correlate
3. Objective intraluminal impedance measurement can be used to distinguish supragastric from gastric belching.

A careful history can help make the diagnosis. Patients are often surprised to learn that belching is not due to gas created in the stomach or intestines; it occurs because the belching comes from swallowed air. The patient's partner, family, or others may observe the air swallowing even if the patient is not aware. Large amounts of belching are more likely due to excessive and uncontrolled supragastric belching, which can occur up to 20 times per minute. If symptoms are troublesome and the technology is available, esophageal impedance/manometry can confirm the diagnosis and help to guide therapy. Patients with supragastric belching do not have increased air in the stomach when an x-ray is taken, but those with gastric belching may show a sizeable gastric air bubble.

***Treatment.***

***Excessive Supragastric Belching.*** It is essential to reassure the patient and explain their symptoms and the mechanism of belching. When the patient discovers they are swallowing excessively, and that the air ingestion leads to the belching, the behavior can reduce. Doctors traditionally recommend dietary or behavioral modification (not sucking candies or chewing gum, eating slowly, encouraging small swallows, and avoiding carbonated beverages). When patients with FD or GERD complain of excessive belching, it seems reasonable to treat these other symptoms first. Successful treatment of excessive belching by a well-informed speech therapist, as well as biofeedback and diaphragmatic breathing training, have been reported to be helpful. The patient should be referred to a mental health provider for evaluation and treatment when there is a suspicion that excessive belching is secondary to a psychiatric disorder. Regardless of the presence of a psychiatric disorder, employing stress-reduction techniques is often helpful.

***Excessive Gastric Belching.*** Acute and severe episodes of gastric belching are rare and occur mainly in mentally challenged patients. Such events can result in the organ twisting on itself (volvulus), as well as obstruction and breathing difficulties, because of increased abdominal pressure. In this case, placing a nasogastric tube to relieve gastric air is one treatment, and sedatives may help to reduce repetitive air swallowing. Patients with chronic gastric belching should avoid carbonated beverages and eat slowly. Treatment with speech therapy to minimize air swallowing seems reasonable. Diaphragmatic breathing may be helpful. Baclofen is a medication that reduces the frequency of LES relaxations and suppresses the swallowing rate. It may help both gastric and supragastric belching events. Surface tension-reducing drugs, such as activated charcoal or simethicone, might prevent gas formation in the intestines and may be tried to reduce symptoms. However, limited scientific evidence is available to support their benefit.

## B3. Nausea/Vomiting Disorders

Nausea is the sensation of an imminent need to vomit; vomiting is the forceful expulsion of gastric or intestinal content through the mouth. These disorders may occur with nausea and vomiting or nausea alone. Rumination (repetitive regurgitation) and regurgitation are effortless and are not associated with nausea or retching, so they are not consistent with this diagnosis (see B4). In Rome IV, we combine nausea and vomiting into a single disorder, Chronic Nausea Vomiting Syndrome (CNVS). We also identify Cyclical Vomiting Syndrome (CVS), which is more episodic, and Cannabinoid Hyperemesis Syndrome (CHS), which is associated with cannabis use. Chronic nausea and vomiting are common symptoms found with many other medical diseases. Therefore, the doctor needs to exclude other diagnoses, such as the constant use of certain medications (e.g., opioids), chronic pain disorders, autonomic neuropathic diseases (e.g., Postural Orthostatic Tachycardia Syndrome, abbreviated as POTS), chronic inflammatory conditions such as inflammatory bowel disease or inflammation of other organs), brain disorders (including brain tumors), and psychiatric disorders such as anxiety and depressive disorders, among others. For further information, go to **http://bit.ly/2wW5hiD**.

**B3a. Chronic Nausea Vomiting Syndrome (CNVS)** – often presents as nausea without vomiting, but when it is severe, vomiting also occurs and is always associated with nausea. Symptoms may occur at any time of day and often with eating, but not always. The clinician must exclude eating disorders and regurgitation (i.e., vomiting without nausea).

**B3b. Cyclical Vomiting Syndrome (CVS)** – characteristically presents as discrete episodes of severe nausea, vomiting, and retching not related to eating. The episodes last for hours to days at a time and then disappear completely.

CVS is often associated with migraine headaches, or the patient may have a family history of migraine. Some patients may have abdominal pain with the CVS episodes; those who have episodes of abdominal pain without vomiting may have abdominal migraine. Notably, many patients find relief by taking baths or showers. Patients with CVS symptoms who use cannabis are diagnosed to have CHS (B3c below).

**B3c. Cannabinoid Hyperemesis Syndrome (CHS)** – a new diagnosis related to increased use of cannabis. In some patients, continued and frequent use of cannabis can produce this syndrome. The clinical features are very much the same as CVS. However, stopping the use of cannabis usually leads to resolution of symptoms (**https://romedross.video/2FtbM1H**).

***Pathophysiology.*** The physiological findings associated with CNVS, CVS, and CHS are challenging to understand. However, these syndromes are different from gastroparesis since they do not have delayed gastric emptying. CNVS may occur with psychological distress or behavioral conditioning. In CVS, dysregulation of the autonomic nervous system occurs. Attacks of CVS also share some features with migraines (and are sometimes mistaken for migraines). These features include the episodic nature of the attacks, intervening periods of wellness, a stereotypic onset of episodes, and associated paleness, hypersensitivity, and fatigue. Other conditions that are sometimes confused with nausea and vomiting syndromes include food allergies and intolerances. CHS is associated with cannabis use. However, some cannabinoids counteract nausea and vomiting, while others may contribute to recurrent vomiting, depending on the dosage. Psychological difficulties present in some patients with nausea and vomiting disorders, and anxiety and depression are more common in adults with any of these conditions.

*Clinical Evaluation.*

**Rome IV Criteria for Nausea and Vomiting Disorders (B3)**

**B3a: Chronic Nausea and Vomiting Syndrome (CNVS)**

Must include all of the following:

1. Bothersome (i.e., severe enough to impact on usual activities) nausea, occurring at least 1 day per week and/or one or more vomiting episodes per week
2. Self-induced vomiting, eating disorders, regurgitation, or rumination are excluded
3. No evidence of organic, systemic, or metabolic diseases that is likely to explain the symptoms on routine investigations (including at upper endoscopy)

---

**B3b: Cyclic Vomiting Syndrome (CVS)**

Must include all of the following:

1. Stereotypical episodes of vomiting regarding onset (acute) and duration (less than 1 week)
2. Three or more discrete episodes in the prior year and two episodes in the past 6 months, occurring at least 1 week apart
3. Absence of vomiting between episodes, but other milder symptoms can be present between cycles

*Supportive criteria:*

History or family history of migraine headaches

---

**B3c: Cannabinoid Hyperemesis Syndrome (CHS)**

Must include all of the following:

1. Stereotypical episodic vomiting resembling cyclic vomiting syndrome (CVS) in terms of onset, duration, and frequency
2. Presentation after prolonged excessive cannabis use
3. Relief of vomiting episodes by sustained cessation of cannabis use

*Supportive criteria:*

May be associated with pathologic bathing behavior (prolonged hot baths or showers)

Nausea and vomiting can result from other gastrointestinal and non-gastrointestinal disorders that must be excluded. Other digestive disorders include gastroparesis, gastric or bowel obstruction, inflammatory bowel disease, and gastric or duodenal ulcers or tumors. Non-gastrointestinal causes include diseases of the brain (e.g., tumors or vascular malformations), metabolic disorders such as uncontrolled diabetes, chronic infection, and advanced cancer. Generally, when the symptoms are acute (happening for the first time or suddenly), a more extensive evaluation is needed. However, according to the definition of this diagnosis, nausea and vomiting symptoms have been present for over 6 months and are chronic, so the focus is more on treatment. Nevertheless, certain laboratory studies need to be done the first time a patient is seen with these symptoms, even if the symptoms have been present for several months. These include blood studies for anemia, liver chemistry tests, and lipase to evaluate for pancreaticobiliary disease (i.e., disorders of the gall bladder, biliary ducts, and pancreas), as well as an upper endoscopy to assess for stomach or duodenal ulcers, obstruction, or tumors.

***Treatment.*** Anti-emetics (i.e., drugs to reduce nausea and prevent vomiting), including Zofran (ondansetron) or Phenergan (promethazine), will often be effective for nausea and vomiting disorders. They are prescribed as needed up to three or four times a day. Antidepressants such as Remeron (mirtazapine) is prescribed for chronic preventative treatment, due to its anti-emetic effect. For CVS, anti-emetics, e.g., Phenergan (promethazine) or Zofran (ondansetron), along with rehydration, are used for acute episodes. To prevent episodes, neuromodulators such as Remeron (mirtazapine) or Zyprexa (olanzapine) provide benefit in reducing nausea and vomiting. At times, anticonvulsants such as Keppra (levetiracetam) or Zonegran (zonisamide) may prevent episodes of CVS. The best treatment for CHS is withdrawal from cannabis use.

## B4. Rumination Syndrome

"Rumination" may bring to mind the reverse peristalsis seen in cows (also called "ruminants") who regurgitate and chew cud from the stomach. Or one may think of the psychological term related to mulling over thoughts. However, Rumination Syndrome (B4) as a DGBI is something very different: it is the repetitive, effortless regurgitation of recently ingested food into the mouth followed by rechewing and re-swallowing or expulsion of the food bolus. This behavior was first reported in the Middle Ages when wandering entertainers would swallow various objects and bring them up upon request. Now, this behavior as a clinical disorder is rarely recognized. I have found that many doctors misdiagnose this syndrome as vomiting or esophageal reflux disease. However, careful attention to the unique clinical features will lead to the diagnosis. For further information on this syndrome see **https://theromefoundation.org/q-a-rumination-2/**.

***Pathophysiology.*** Rumination occurs when the lower esophageal sphincter (LES), the muscle separating the esophagus from the stomach, relaxes at the same time that the diaphragm contracts rhythmically, thereby increasing intra-abdominal pressure. Increased abdominal pressure forces the contents in the stomach to go up through the LES and the esophagus and then into the mouth. At this point, the patient will re-chew the food and swallow it or spit it out. This disorder was first reportedly clinically in mentally challenged children, where it was considered a self-stimulation habit. In adults, Rumination Syndrome may occur along with psychological difficulties. Stressful life events may trigger symptom onset in some patients. Rumination can also be associated with eating disorders such as bulimia nervosa, where the food is more commonly expelled rather than re-swallowed.

### *Clinical Evaluation.*

**Rome IV Criteria for Rumination Syndrome (B4)**

Must include all of the following:

1. Persistent or recurrent regurgitation of recently ingested food into the mouth with subsequent spitting or re-mastication and swallowing
2. Regurgitation is not preceded by retching

*Supportive criteria:*

1. Effortless regurgitation events are usually not preceded by nausea
2. Regurgitant contains recognizable food that might have a pleasant taste
3. The process tends to cease when the regurgitated material becomes acidic

Episodes or rumination can occur on occasion or be present with every meal. There is no nausea retching or forceful expulsion as with vomiting. The regurgitation can begin within a few minutes of eating, and it commonly stops when the food turns sour or bitter tasting from stomach acid. Weight loss can occur, particularly when associated with an eating disorder. Heartburn with esophageal erosions may be present, but this is due to the regurgitation rather than to GERD per se. Doctors need to exclude other diagnoses such as GERD, gastroparesis, achalasia, bowel obstruction, or Functional Nausea/Vomiting Syndrome. Upper endoscopy and esophageal manometry can demonstrate the typical findings that confirm this diagnosis. However, a careful history is often sufficient to make the diagnosis.

***Treatment.*** Lifestyle, medication, surgical, and behavioral therapies lead to variable degrees of success with Rumination Syndrome. Gum chewing may help children with rumination. Proton pump inhibitors such as Nexium (esomeprazole) or Prilosec (omeprazole) are prescribed to suppress heartburn and protect the esophageal mucosa during regurgitations. The medication Baclofen may reduce the frequency of rumination episodes preventing LES relaxations. The mainstay of treatment for Rumination Syndrome involves behavioral modification. Diaphragmatic breathing is one form of behavioral modification that reduces the urge to regurgitate and also has a relaxing effect.[26] It is easy to learn the method, as demonstrated in this video: **https://romedross.video/3azBfEE**. Hiatal hernia surgery (Nissen fundoplication) has been proposed for those who don't respond to these treatments.

## C. Bowel Disorders[18]

Functional bowel disorders are very prevalent and can affect all ages and members of society. The most frequently experienced symptoms include abdominal pain (usually in the lower abdomen), diarrhea, constipation, and bloating (in any combination). Irritable Bowel Syndrome (IBS), which requires the presence of abdominal pain together with irregular bowel habit, and Functional Constipation (FC) are the most common functional bowel disorders, and symptoms may overlap or alternate in time (see below). Less common bowel disorders are Functional Diarrhea, Functional Abdominal Bloating, and Opioid-Induced Constipation. Patient-specific differences in quantity, intensity, frequency, and severity of the symptoms characterize each of these disorders.

The use of diagnostic criteria is essential for research to separate the different disorders for investigation. In clinical practice, however, the subgroups described below are not necessarily distinguishable as discrete entities, and treatments overlap. For example, the sub-group of IBS patients with predominant constipation (IBS-C) overlaps with those that have Functional Constipation, and IBS-D overlaps with those that have Functional Diarrhea. The difference lies in the presence and impact of pain. In IBS-C and IBS-D, pain is the predominant symptom, while in Functional Constipation or Functional Diarrhea, pain is absent or only secondary. Unfortunately, many doctors are not familiar with the Rome criteria and assume that all patients within these categories just have IBS or that it's "functional," meaning psychiatric or untreatable. This common error can impair diagnostic decision making and implementation of appropriate, well-targeted treatments.

### C1. Irritable Bowel Syndrome (IBS)

While IBS is not the most common of the DGBI, it is the one that most patients, doctors, and the media recognize. However, inappropriately diagnosing all bowel disorders as IBS may affect proper treatment. When correctly identified, IBS is a functional bowel disorder in which recurrent abdominal pain is related to defecation. Disordered bowel habits, such as constipation, diarrhea, or a mixture of both, are typically present, as are symptoms of abdominal bloating and distension. **To meet the diagnostic criteria for IBS, the following need to be present: pain related to defecation, on average at least 1 day a week in the past 3 months, associated with a change in frequency of stool and a change in the form (appearance) of stool.** According to the predominant bowel habit—based upon stool form on days with at least one abnormal bowel movement—IBS is sub-classified into four main subtypes:

- **C1a. IBS with predominant constipation (IBS-C)**
- **C1b. IBS with predominant diarrhea (IBS-D)**
- **C1c. IBS with mixed bowel habits (IBS-M)**
- **C1d. IBS with unspecified bowel habits (IBS-U)**

The Bristol Stool Form Scale (BSFS), shown in Figure 12 below, is used to identify the predominant stool pattern. https://romedross.video/Q_A_IBSCD.

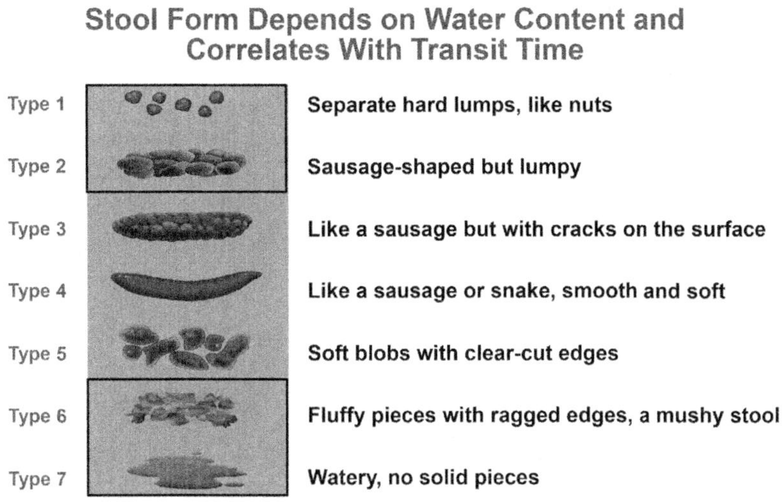




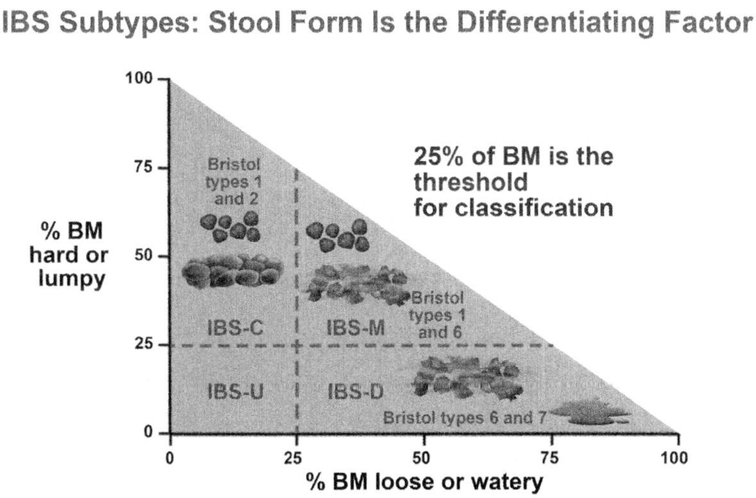




Figure 12. **Bristol Stool Form Scale (BSFS)** and its use to diagnose diarrhea and constipation. The BSFS is a useful tool to evaluate bowel habit; it is a reliable surrogate marker for colonic transit. IBS subtypes should be classified to stool consistency, using the BSFS. IBS subtyping is more accurate when patients have at least 4 days of abnormal bowel habits per month. Bowel habit subtypes should be based on BSFS for days with abnormal bowel habits.[18]

Using the BSFS (in which > represents "more than" and < represents "less than"), the four types of IBS subtypes are classified as follows:

**IBS with Predominant Constipation (IBS-C):** > ¼ (25%) of bowel movements with Bristol stool types 1 or 2 and < ¼ (25%) of bowel movements with Bristol stool types 6 or 7. Alternatively, the patient reports that abnormal bowel movements are usually constipation (like types 1 or 2 in the picture of BSF).

**IBS with Predominant Diarrhea (IBS-D):** > ¼ (25%) of bowel movements with Bristol stool types 6 or 7 and < ¼ (25%) of bowel movements with Bristol stool types 1 or 2. Alternatively, the patient reports that abnormal bowel movements are usually diarrhea (like types 6 or 7 in the picture of BSF).

**IBS with Mixed Bowel Habits (IBS-M):** > ¼ (25%) of bowel movements with Bristol stool types 1 or 2 and > ¼ (25%) of bowel movements with Bristol stool types 6 or 7. Alternatively, the patient reports that abnormal bowel movements are usually both constipation and diarrhea (more than ¼ of all the abnormal bowel movements were constipation, and more than ¼ were diarrhea, using the picture of BSF).

**IBS Unclassified (IBS-U):** Patients who meet diagnostic criteria for IBS but whose bowel habits cannot be accurately categorized into one of the three groups above have IBS-U. Alternatively, the patient reports that abnormal stools (both diarrhea and constipation) are rare.

***Pathophysiology.*** Multiple factors can lead to the symptoms of IBS. Genetic, environmental, and psychosocial factors can increase the risk of developing it. Factors that trigger the onset or flare-up of IBS symptoms include prior gastroenteritis (i.e., post-infection IBS), food intolerances, hormonal changes (such as menses, chronic stress), and other psychological factors, including early trauma. Symptoms result from any combination of altered GI motility, visceral hypersensitivity, increased intestinal permeability, immune activation of the bowel mucosa, alteration in the microbiota, and disturbances in brain-gut function.

***Clinical Evaluation.***

**Rome IV Criteria for Irritable Bowel Syndrome (C1)**

Recurrent abdominal pain, on average, at least 1 day per week, associated with two or more of the following criteria:

1. Related to defecation
2. Associated with a change in frequency of stool
3. Associated with a change in form (appearance) of stool

To fulfill the diagnosis of IBS, a patient needs to meet the Rome IV criteria and must not have any other medical disorders that may produce the same symptoms. A medical history should include whether the symptoms developed after a GI infection. A dietary assessment includes reviewing the food components that affect bowel habits and possibly aggravate IBS symptoms (with attention to the intake of dairy products, wheat, gluten, caffeine, fruit, vegetables, juices, sweetened soft drinks, and chewing gum). A brief psychosocial review should assess psychological factors, major life events, and the presence of psychiatric disease, particularly anxiety and depression. A thorough physical exam should include the abdomen to evaluate for bowel sounds, abnormal physical findings, and areas of tenderness. A digital rectal examination excludes external hemorrhoids and rectal masses and determines if the sphincter is weak or fails to relax completely. Diagnostic testing and blood studies may be needed to rule out celiac disease or inflammatory bowel disease, depending on the findings. In older patients, this usually requires a colonoscopy. Patients with IBS may also have other co-existing GI and non-GI symptoms. These may include functional dyspepsia, headache, fatigue, fibromyalgia, and pelvic floor disorders, all of which may need further evaluation and concurrent treatment.

The diagnostic evaluation needs to consider many factors. For example, younger patients whose symptoms are recent and mild may receive less evaluation than older patients or patients with other clinical findings. When alarm signs or "red flags" are present, the doctor will more likely consider additional testing. Red flags can include (a) rectal bleeding or positive occult blood in the stool, (b) iron deficiency anemia, (c) weight loss, (d) family history of colon cancer or inflammatory bowel disease, (e) abnormal physical examination or laboratory studies, (f) fever, or (g) age over 50 years. When any of these is present, the doctor will likely schedule a colonoscopy or other studies, including a CT scan, stool testing, and other blood studies. Also, diagnostic studies will differ depending on whether diarrhea or constipation predominates. With diarrhea, the doctor may do a colonoscopy and take biopsies to exclude microscopic colitis, or even do an upper endoscopy and biopsy to identify celiac disease. With constipation, the doctor may evaluate the speed of colonic evacuation using a stool marker transit test or an anorectal motility test. Once this evaluation is complete, the next step is to focus on management. If the patient later experiences a new type of pain, weight loss, or has an abnormal physical examination or new laboratory findings, diagnostic studies need to be repeated.

***Treatment.*** IBS treatment begins by explaining the condition, providing reassurance that it is benign, and educating the patient about the utility and safety of diagnostic tests and treatment options. The cornerstone for effective therapy is the patient-doctor relationship; with this in place, IBS is more specifically managed, based on the type and severity of symptoms and the nature of associated psychosocial issues. As scary as pain, diarrhea, and other symptoms seem to be, doctors must convey that these symptoms do not represent a severe illness. Undue worry may worsen how symptoms are experienced and lead to as much distress as the symptoms themselves. This may also lead to unjustified and even hazardous investigations and procedures. Calm the brain, calm the gut.

Lifestyle modifications such as exercise, stress reduction, and attention to disturbed sleep may improve IBS symptoms. Supplementing dietary fiber may be considered for milder forms of IBS-C, but insoluble fiber, and particularly bran, can exacerbate problems of abdominal distention and flatulence.

Let's address how diet can help or not help. For patients with IBS-D in particular, a low FODMAP (an acronym for fermentable oligosaccharides, disaccharides, monosaccharides, and polyols, which include sugar alcohols such as sorbitol, mannitol, xylitol, and maltitol) diet is associated with reduced fermentation in the gut and improved symptoms. This occurs because these poorly absorbed food substances are broken down by bacteria to produce gas, which increases symptoms of pain, bloating, and diarrhea. Dietary limitation of wheat, fructans, or gluten may improve symptoms in some IBS patients. However, these items are also part of a low FODMAP diet and won't help if the FODMAP diet is not successful. Dietary restriction can help to identify trigger foods, so if certain food items do not lead to symptoms, they should no longer be restricted. A therapeutic trial restricting any of these substances may be considered. However, in my practice, I also see patients who continue low FODMAP diets or gluten restriction, even when they see no benefit. Patients undergoing dietary restriction trials need medical or dietary guidance. This is done first to see if restriction achieves any benefit. Without benefit, these diets should be abandoned. If symptoms improve with FODMAP restriction, some foods should be reintroduced so that the diet is only limited to those foods that cause symptoms.

Sometimes I see patients who excessively restrict food to the point of developing nutritional difficulties. Over-restriction can occur when eating causes pain, so patients reduce the amount they eat to avoid pain. This is called "sitophobia" (fear of eating). Others over-restrict the types of foods they eat because they think that certain foods that are "unhealthy" are producing their symptoms. This is called "orthorexia." Another group may severely restrict the quantity of food and may become malnourished. This is called Avoidance Restrictive Food Intake Disorders (ARFID) and is a type of eating disorder. These behaviors are based on efforts by patients to exert control over their symptoms. However, the doctor needs to determine which patients can be managed effectively by adjusting their diet and medication, and which patients also require assistance from a mental health specialist to reframe dysfunctional thinking and eating behaviors.

With milder symptoms, patients with IBS can, on occasion, increase fiber, take Miralax or Glycolax (PEG solution) or OTC laxatives if they have IBS-C, and Imodium (loperamide) if they have IBS-D. Antispasmodic medications such as Bentyl (dicyclomine) or Levsin (hyoscyamine) can reduce abdominal pain, especially if the pain occurs after eating. Over-the-counter products or "medical foods," including peppermint oil (e.g., IBSGard), Enterogram (bovine serum globulin), human milk oligosaccharide (Holigos), and pre- and probiotics may also be helpful.

L-Glutamine is another OTC product that is being used to stabilize the barrier of the lining of the gut (i.e., to treat "leaky gut").

Prescription medications are used when symptoms are more severe or if changes in lifestyle and the addition of OTC products or dietary measures are not sufficient. The type of medication will depend on the type and severity of symptoms. For abdominal bloating or IBS-D with bloating, a poorly absorbable antibiotic Xifaxan (rifaximin) could be considered. For IBS-C, secretagogues such as Linzess (linaclotide), Amitiza (lubiprostone), Trulance (plecanatide), or a prokinetic agent that stimulates the bowel, such as Zelnorm (tegaserod), have all shown benefit for pain and constipation. With IBS-D, Viberzi (eluxadoline), Lotronex (alosetron), Questran (cholestyramine), Zofran (ondansetron), and Xifaxan (rifaximin) may be tried.

Neuromodulators are prescribed when pain is severe or when associated symptoms of anxiety or depression occur with the symptoms. These may include a tricyclic antidepressant (TCA), such as Elavil (amitriptyline), Pamelor (nortriptyline), or Norpramin (desipramine), especially when diarrhea is present; or selective norepinephrine, a serotonin reuptake inhibitor (SNRI), such as Cymbalta (duloxetine).

Finally, psychological treatments such as cognitive-behavioral therapy (CBT), hypnotherapy, and mindfulness meditation have been shown effective for most patients with IBS. Their benefit is additive to medical treatments, and they demonstrate sustained effectiveness even after the treatment period is completed.[27]

## C2. Functional Constipation (FC)

While many will assume that constipation means infrequent bowel movements, Functional Constipation (FC), also called Chronic Idiopathic Constipation (CIC), relates to symptoms of difficult, infrequent, or incomplete defecation. The number of bowel movements each day may be normal (normal is three bowel movements a week to three a day). Still, other symptoms relating to the effort to evacuate or a sense of not having finished are common. Bloating is also a common feature. Although FC is much like IBS-C, pain is not a dominant feature.

***Pathophysiology.*** Symptoms of FC arise for a variety of reasons. There is some evidence that it tends to run in families, but there is little evidence of any direct genetic cause. A few pediatric studies suggest that lifestyle factors in childhood (low-fiber intake, low fluid intake, and ignoring the call to stool) may lead to the later development of constipation. High-fiber intake and regular exercise are associated with less constipation, but increasing fluid intake shows no benefit. Psychological and behavioral features like stress, anxiety, and early toilet training can affect constipation, stool output, and the motility of the gut.

Functional Constipation is comprised of three main categories: (a) normal-transit constipation, (b) slow-transit constipation where different colonic segments may be affected, and (c) defecatory or rectal evacuation disorders. Slow-transit constipation can be evaluated by ingesting radiopaque (e.g., Sitzmark, Intramarx) markers and determining how many markers are retained in the colon after a certain number of days. About one-third of patients have a rectal evacuation disorder. They report straining and difficulty evacuating the stool. This is called Dyssynergic Defecation, or pelvic floor dyssynergia, and results from incomplete relaxation of the levator (pelvic floor) muscles, or inadequate rectal propulsion, causing a type of blockage. The diagnosis can be made by rectal examination and confirmed by anorectal motility testing.

Most FC patients do not show visceral hypersensitivity, as seen with IBS. Still, some have rectal hyposensitivity (abnormally low sensitivity of the rectum), and some show impairment in the autonomic nervous system and other changes, such as reduced neurotransmitter levels and fewer interstitial cells (cells that lie in the spaces between the functional cells in the colon).

***Clinical Evaluation.***

**Rome IV Criteria for Functional Constipation (FC) (C2)**

1. Must include two or more of the following:
   a. Straining during more than one-fourth (25%) of defecations
   b. Lumpy or hard stools more than one-fourth (25%) of defecations
   c. Sensation of incomplete evacuation more than one-fourth (25%) of defecations
   d. Sensation of anorectal obstruction/blockage during more than one-fourth (25%) of defecations
   e. Manual maneuvers to facilitate more than one-fourth (25%) of defecations (e.g., digital evacuation, support of the pelvic floor by "splinting" maneuvers)
   f. Fewer than three spontaneous bowel movements per week
2. Loose stools are rarely present without the use of laxatives)
3. Insufficient criteria for irritable bowel syndrome

A survey of patients with FC found that the most frequent symptoms were straining (79%), hard stools (71%), abdominal discomfort (62%), bloating (57%), infrequent bowel movements (57%), and feelings of incomplete evacuation (54%). Other medical factors may cause secondary constipation (primary constipation means no other cause is identified). These factors causing secondary constipation include a very low-fiber diet, medications including opioids, antispasmodics, tricyclic antidepressants, anti-seizure drugs, and calcium channel blockers used for high blood pressure. Other medical diseases may also cause constipation, including colorectal cancer, Parkinson's disease, diverticular disease, and endocrine disorders like hypothyroidism. Constipation is also more common in the elderly.

Patients may misperceive that their bowel pattern is constipation. Some believe they have constipation when they don't have a bowel movement every day; it is also normal to have a bowel movement every other day or even twice a week. Straining with defecation, even when occurring every day, may suggest Dyssynergic Defecation (see anorectal disorders). This requires additional evaluation and treatment. Some patients report constipation when they have abdominal discomfort and "can't go," even if the stool has not yet reached the rectum. Therefore, a detailed history should include the duration of symptoms, the presence and frequency of bowel movements, stool consistency (using the Bristol Stool Form Scale), the presence of abdominal pain, bloating or distension, and any difficulty with evacuation (including straining, a sense of an incomplete passage, and efforts to remove the stool).

The physical examination should include an abdominal examination to assess whether fecal material is being retained in the colon, and a pelvic and rectal exam to determine if there is incomplete pelvic floor relaxation or if a rectocele is present. The presence of alarm signs might lead to further evaluation. These include recent onset of severe constipation, unintentional weight loss (>10% in 3 months), rectal bleeding (in the absence of documented bleeding hemorrhoids or anal fissures), and a family history of colon cancer or polyposis syndromes. Finally, if the patient has difficulty evacuating (Dyssynergic Defecation), an anorectal motility study and balloon expulsion test can confirm pelvic floor dyssynergia, and on occasion, a defecogram done by CT or barium can identify other pelvic floor problems, such as an enterocele or rectocele that is causing a difficult evacuation.

The diagnosis is made when the Rome IV criteria are met, there are no alarm signs, and when other diagnostic possibilities have been excluded. However, in an older patient or in someone who has newly developed constipation, a colonoscopy is required to rule out the possibility that other medical diseases are causing these symptoms.

***Treatment.*** Treatment should begin by educating the patient about FC and eliminating medications that can cause or worsen constipation. The diet should contain an adequate amount of fiber. It helps to schedule a routine bathroom time (after the morning or evening meal), elevating the feet, if need be, with a footstool (e.g., "squatty potty") or by using a toilet that is lower to the ground. Treatment can begin with a high-fiber diet or fiber supplement (e.g., Metamucil, Citrucel). Occasional use of "osmotic" laxatives (e.g., lactulose, mannitol, and sorbitol), which are not absorbed by the small intestine and accelerate transit by increasing the mass of the stool and stimulating secretion and motility, can be considered. Saline laxatives (magnesium citrate, magnesium sulfate, sodium, and disodium phosphate) induce movement of water into the small intestine and colon; these should be used cautiously in older people and anyone with kidney problems. Miralax or Glycolax (PEG solution) is safe, and the single daily dose can be titrated to higher levels when symptoms are more severe. Stimulant laxatives (bisacodyl, sodium picosulfate, cascara sagrada, aloe, and senna) stimulate intestinal motility. They can occasionally be used for "rescue"—i.e., if an individual being treated for constipation has not had a bowel movement after 3 or more days. We do not recommend this for daily use.

When the patient has not responded to diet or over-the-counter medications, they may need prescription medicines. Secretagogues increase fluid into the intestines to produce a more frequent, softer stool, and to reduce bloating. These medications include Amitiza (lubiprostone), Linzess (linaclotide), and Trulance (plecanatide). Prokinetics are promotility medications that increase the transit rate of stool through the colon. These include Motegrity (prucalopride) or Zelnorm (tegaserod). When there is difficulty evacuating due to incomplete relaxation of the pelvic floor muscles (Dyssynergic Defecation), anorectal biofeedback is the treatment of choice. See this video on Dyssynergic Defecation: **https://romedross.video/Q_A_DysynDefecConstip** and also go to the section on Anorectal Disorders.

## C3. Functional Diarrhea (FDr)

This disorder is characterized by usually painless loose or watery stools occurring at least 25% of the time. Abdominal pain or bothersome bloating are typically absent, but if present is mild. Therefore, these patients do not have IBS-D, where the pain is dominant.

***Pathophysiology.*** As with other DGBI, no single pathophysiological abnormality can explain the cause of FDr in every patient. Altered motility of the GI system, brain-gut disturbances, genetic and environmental factors, prior infections (leading to post-infectious FDr), and psychosocial factors may all contribute. Increased gastrointestinal motility is thought to be the leading cause of FDr, with evidence for increased colonic propagating and decreased non-propagating contractions (propagated contractions work to push feces through the colon). This leads to more rapid transit through the colon and less absorption of fluid, leading to liquid or loose stools.

***Clinical Evaluation.***

**Rome IV Criteria for Functional Diarrhea (C3)**

Must include both of the following:

1. Loose or watery stools, without predominant abdominal pain or bothersome bloating, occurring in >25% of stools
2. Patients meeting criteria for diarrhea-predominant IBS should be excluded

Diagnosis of FDr is based on a carefully taken clinical history, physical examination, and limited diagnostic tests. The patient's diarrhea is defined by stool *form*, not stool frequency. It can be helpful to keep a stool diary, using the BSFS, to identify the proportion of types 6 and 7 (see Figure 12). A dietary history should exclude symptoms from excess lactose and fructose and to make sure that the patient is not eating excess amounts of poorly absorbed carbohydrates, such as beans and legumes. Alarm features if present should prompt further investigation. These features include unintentional weight loss, diarrhea that wakes up the patient, recent antibiotic use, blood in the stool (if no bleeding hemorrhoids or anal fissures are present), a high volume of diarrhea, very frequent bowel movements (>6–10 per day), evidence of malnutrition, or a family history of colorectal neoplasia, celiac disease, or inflammatory bowel disease.

The physical examination should be normal. An anorectal examination should be performed to assess anal sphincter tone (especially important in patients with incontinence or Dyssynergic Defecation); and to identify any mass, fissure, or hemorrhoids that may be present (especially important in patients with hematochezia). Blood studies, including a CBC and C-reactive protein, are usually ordered in all patients with chronic diarrhea, and if hyperthyroidism is suspected a thyroid panel should be obtained. A tissue transglutaminase (TTG) blood test determines if celiac disease is present. Stool analysis should evaluate white cells, calprotectin if there is clinical suspicion of inflammatory bowel disease (IBD), and fecal elastase to exclude pancreatic malabsorption. With high-volume diarrhea, a 24-hour stool collection will determine increased volume, the presence of increased fat (suggesting malabsorption), and laxatives. A colonoscopy is done for patients who have failed to benefit from empiric therapy, in those with alarm symptoms, and in all patients older than age 50. Random biopsies should be obtained from both the right and left colon to rule out microscopic colitis.

***Treatment.*** Treatment for FDr patients is mainly empiric and arises from studies of patients with other conditions, such as IBS-D. Dietary changes and fiber supplements have not sufficiently been evaluated. Loperamide (an opioid) improves stool frequency and consistency, as well as urgency and incontinence, in patients with FDr and IBS-D. Questran (cholestyramine) is effective and safe for short-term treatment of patients when FDr is secondary to bile acid malabsorption. Antibiotics such as Xifaxan (rifaximin) and 5-HT3 antagonists such as Lotronex (alosetron) or Zofran (ondansetron) may all improve diarrhea symptoms but have not been tested specifically in FDr patients. There is also little data on psychological treatments for FDr. However, because diarrhea can be a physiological stress response and anxiety may be associated, this type of therapy is logical.

## C4. Functional Abdominal Bloating/Distension (FAB/FAD)

This disorder is characterized by recurrent symptoms of abdominal fullness, pressure, or a sensation of trapped gas (i.e., bloating – FAB), or a measurable increase in abdominal girth (i.e., distension – FAD) that is not explained by other DGBI. Mild abdominal pain or minor bowel movement abnormalities may co-exist. FAB and FAD may exist independently, but more often they coincide in the same individual. They are therefore classified as a single entity (Functional Abdominal Bloating/Distention), although they encompass two different symptoms/signs.

***Pathophysiology.*** The physiological causes of bloating are not entirely understood, partly because the reasons vary from patient to patient. Potentially, these causes can include visceral hypersensitivity, abnormal transit of gas in the intestine, impaired evacuation of rectal gas, fermentation in the colon, bacterial overgrowth in the small intestine, and changes in the gut microbiota. The pathophysiology of abdominal distention is best understood as an abnormal reflex of the diaphragm and abdominal wall muscles that often, but not always, occurs after eating. The reflex is called abdominophrenic dyssynergia (**https://romedross.video/Q_A_AbdomDyssyn**). It causes the diaphragm to push down and the abdominal rectus muscle to relax, which leads to the distension.[28] It is not related to increased intestinal gas. Also, slow intestinal transit may contribute to distention in some patients.

***Clinical Evaluation.***

**Rome IV Criteria for Functional Bloating/Distension (FAB/FAD) (C4)**

Must include both of the following:

1. Recurrent bloating and/or distention occurring, on average, at least 1 day per week; abdominal bloating and/or distention predominates over other symptoms
2. There are insufficient criteria for a diagnosis of irritable bowel syndrome, functional constipation, functional diarrhea, or postprandial distress syndrome

Mild pain related to bloating may be present as well as minor bowel movement abnormalities

FAB/FAD is diagnosed by taking a clinical history, doing a physical exam, and performing limited diagnostic studies. Evaluation of a patient with abdominal bloating and/or distention should begin with a careful history, including when symptoms began; whether symptoms are present that would suggest other DGBI; and the relationship between diet (wheat, dairy, fructose, fiber, non-absorbable sugars) and bowel habits. Alarm features, including anemia and unintentional weight loss, should be assessed, as they may indicate a malabsorptive process. Symptoms of FAB/FAD usually get worse as the day progresses, particularly after meals, but get better during the overnight. Diurnal (daytime) worsening of bloating is frequently accompanied by increased abdominal girth. The critical point is that the distension is usually not constant; if it is, consider other diagnostic possibilities. During the physical examination, the doctor should check for abdominal distention (a visible increase in abdominal girth). A distended abdomen may be associated with abnormal bowel sounds (increased with obstruction and decreased with ileus), the presence of a mass (e.g., large palpable colon suggesting fecal mass, an enlarged liver, or bowel tumor), and fluid (e.g., ascites). An abdominal x-ray can evaluate for a possible a fecal mass, an obstruction, or a pseudo-obstruction. A CBC will determine if anemia or inflammation is present, and a pelvic examination is required to exclude gynecological causes of distension (e.g., large ovarian cyst or fibroid). Blood tests are ordered to identify celiac disease (TTG), often followed by upper endoscopy with duodenal biopsies; bacterial overgrowth in the small intestine can be evaluated by cultures or a breath test.

***Treatment.*** Few therapeutic trials have been conducted in patients with FAB/FAD. Most studies have evaluated abdominal bloating in patients with other DGBI.

Simethicone and other anti-foaming agents (e.g., Gas-X) or peppermint oil may be tried, but studies are limited. Secretagogues such as Amitiza (lubiprostone), Linzess (linaclotide), and Trulance (plecanatide) have reduced bloating symptoms in patients with IBS-C but have not been tested for FAB/FAD. Neuromodulators, including tricyclic antidepressants such as Pamelor (desipramine), or serotonin-norepinephrine reuptake inhibitors such as Cymbalta (duloxetine), may improve the sensation of bloating. In my experience, neuromodulators can reduce distension from APD by breaking the pain/bloating reflex cycle that leads to the distension. Cognitive-behavioral therapy may be considered, but its effects are still unclear. Neostigmine, a promotility drug, has been shown to clear large amounts of gas. Bloxiverz (neostigmine) and Mestinon (pyridostigmine) can help clear accumulated gas resulting from pseudo-obstruction (where motility is so slow there appears to be a blockage, though this is not the case), but their value with FAB/FAD is not yet determined.

## C6. Opioid-Induced Constipation (OIC)

This is a new category for Rome IV that has become more recognized because of the increased use of opioids in society. It is part of a spectrum of symptoms in the GI tract and the central nervous system. These may overlap with or worsen the symptoms of other DGBI. For example, FC may overlap with or worsen OIC (and vice versa); this is often called opioid associated constipation (OAC).

***Pathophysiology.*** Opioids act on the (mu and delta) opioid chemical receptors of the gut to slow down motility and secretion, so constipation is a common side effect of opioids. Other symptoms resulting from prolonged use of opioids include gastroparesis (where gastric emptying is delayed), intestinal pseudo-obstruction (the entire GI tract is slowed down), and OIC, as discussed here. Nausea and vomiting may also be side effects due to the impact of opioids on nausea centers.

***Clinical Evaluation.***

**Rome IV Criteria for Opioid-Induced Constipation (OIC) (C6)**

1. New or worsening symptoms of constipation when initiating, changing, or increasing opioid therapy that must include two or more of the following:
   a. Straining during more than one-fourth (25%) of defecations
   b. Lumpy or hard stools (BSFS 1–2) more than one-fourth (25%) of defecations
   c. Sensation of incomplete evacuation more than one-fourth (25%) of defecations
   d. Sensation of anorectal obstruction/blockage more than one-fourth (25%) of defecations
   e. Manual maneuvers to facilitate more than one-fourth (25%) of defecations (e.g., digital evacuation, support of the pelvic floor)
   f. Fewer than three spontaneous bowel movements per week
2. Loose stools are rarely present without the use of laxatives

The diagnosis of OIC should be made based on clinical history, physical examination, and limited diagnostic tests and is similar to the evaluation of chronic constipation. The first step, however, is to ascertain whether there is a temporal relationship between constipation symptoms and opioid use (see diagnostic criteria). If such a link does exist, the clinician should identify the type, severity, and frequency of constipation symptoms (e.g., reduced stool frequency, straining, sense of incomplete evacuation, hard stools). The presence of alarm features, such as unintentional weight loss, rectal bleeding (in the absence of documented bleeding hemorrhoids or anal fissures), and a family history of colon cancer (or familial polyposis syndromes) should be obtained. A physical examination determines whether there is significant fecal retention evidenced by fullness in the colon or a structural finding such as an abdominal mass that accounts for symptoms. The anorectal exam evaluates structural issues causing bowel obstruction or incomplete relaxation of the pelvic floor (Dyssynergic Defecation). If indicated, simple laboratory tests (e.g., CBC, complete metabolic profile, serum calcium, and thyroid-stimulating hormone) are reasonable, and an abdominal x-ray (kidney, ureter, and bladder) can identify the impaction of feces and level of stool burden. Patients older than 50 (or 45 and older in African Americans) should have a screening colonoscopy (based on national recommendations), as should patients with warning signs (e.g., anemia, hematochezia not thought due to hemorrhoidal bleeding or fissures, and a family history of colorectal cancer). Patients with OIC report a significant reduction in quality of life.

***Treatment.*** The best treatment would be to stop the opioids. If that is not possible then other options may be considered. If OIC is mild, initial treatment is similar to that of Functional Constipation. Amitiza (lubiprostone) is FDA-approved for the treatment of OIC in adults; Linzess (linaclotide) and Trulance (plecanatide) may also be tried. Additional treatment options for OIC involve the use of a more specific class of medications designated as Peripherally Acting Mu Opioid Receptor Antagonists (PAMORA). These specifically target OIC by blocking or minimizing negative opioid actions on the bowel that affect the intestinal secretion and colonic propulsion, while retaining the central effects on pain. Three such agents are now available: Relistor (methylnaltexone), Movantik (naloxegol) and Symproic (naldemedine).

## D. Centrally Mediated Disorders of Gastrointestinal Pain[19]

### *Historical Perspective on Chronic Abdominal Pain*

To understand Centrally Mediated Disorders of Gastrointestinal Pain, previously called Functional Abdominal Pain Syndrome, we need to take a deeper dive into the origins of the brain-gut axis and its relation to pain. Knowledge of this axis began in the 1940s when Henry Beecher, an anesthesiologist, studied soldiers wounded in battle during WWII. He found that at the time of the injury, the soldiers reported little or no pain and required no morphine. Later at the hospital, however, the pain and their need for morphine increased. Beecher presumed that while at the battlefront, an injury led to the high expectation of going back to safety: it was a "ticket to the hospital" and security. This positive expectation created an emotional component that blocked the effect of the injury on the pain experience. Later work by psychologists Melzack and Wall[29] confirmed that pain results not only from the nerves in the injured part of the body sending signals to the brain. Instead, there is a bidirectional system in which the brain can also modify nerve messages from the body going to the brain by way of a spinal cord "gate." In other words, mental and emotional factors influence the *experience* of the pain by reducing signals coming to the brain. Their research led to the creation of the Gate Control Theory first published in 1965, for which Melzack and Wall received the Nobel Prize in Physiology. If you like, you may view this video explanation: **https://romedross.video/Brain-GutAxis**.

Let's consider some real-life examples. Imagine that you are running a race and sprain your ankle. Your focused attention on the competition may block the pain signals coming from the nerves in your ankle, and you might not experience the pain until after the race. People say this is due to "adrenaline," which is correct. Norepinephrine (similar to adrenaline) is the neurotransmitter that blocks brain signals going to the brain from the body. Conversely, studies show that when you experience severe stress, the brain may send messages down to the spinal cord to "open the gate," leading to increased throughput of nerve signals to the brain, and higher pain experience, even if there is little or no injury. Also, hypnosis can reduce pain, or it can induce pain from the suggested part of the body. Therefore, we have learned that the brain-gut axis, gate-control pathway has a "switch" mechanism, as shown in Figure 13. Pain signals that arise in the gut go to the brain, yet the brain can reciprocally send nerve signals to the gut to block (downregulate) or even enhance (upregulate) the pain experience.

### *From Acute to Chronic Pain*

So how can we explain the origins of chronic abdominal pain, especially when all the GI studies are negative? Now we have the answer. The degree to which the brain and gut are interacting determines the gastrointestinal pain experience occurring through the brain-gut axis. When we have a bowel infection or bowel blockage, the

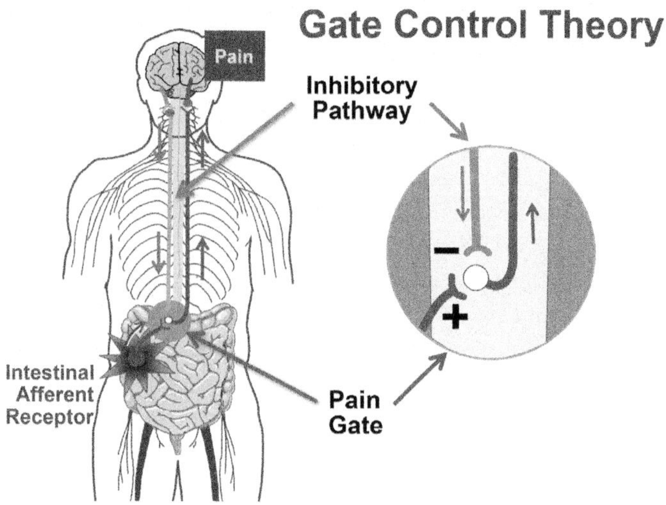


**Figure 13.** Gate control theory. This image demonstrates the brain-gut axis and the gate-control mechanism for GI pain. Pain that begins in the gut ascends to the dorsal horn of the spinal cord. Then, second-order neurons go to the midbrain and limbic structures. Finally, third-order neurons go to the cortex (e.g., cingulate cortex and other areas) where the pain is experienced. The gate control theory of pain explains the brain's ability to reciprocally facilitate or block ("gate") the ascending signal from the dorsal horn going to the brain, thereby heightening or reducing the experience of the pain. This can occur by distraction, focused attention, meditation, hypnosis, or medications like neuromodulators. Chronic GI pain results from dysregulation of this brain-gut pathway. With visceral hypersensitivity there is increased nerve activity going from the GI tract to the spinal cord and brain. Then at the spinal cord there is greater activity going to the brain as well as a failure of the brain to sufficiently block or downregulate the ascending signal at the dorsal horn of the cord (central hypersensitivity). The use of neuromodulators and behavioral treatments can help reset this dysregulated system and reduce pain. For a full discussion go to: **https://romedross.video/Brain-GutAxis**.

nerve signals are very active at the gut level, and most of the pain experience arises from the disease, injury, or an infection. This is acute pain, and treating the GI injury removes the pain.

Chronic abdominal pain is something different. Clinically, I often see patients who develop GI pain that begins as occasional or infrequent episodes, but over time the pain becomes severe and constant. We say that they develop chronic abdominal pain, and it occurs via the gate-control mechanism. We know that severe emotional distress lowers the pain threshold, and the sensation of pain increases; in effect, stress "upregulates" even low-level nerve signals producing more pain. We also know that when the nerve signals from the gut repeatedly go to the spinal cord, the nerves in the spinal cord amplify the signals going to the brain. We call this the "wind-up" phenomenon. In this way, a vicious cycle ensues: as more pain signals go to the brain, pain severity increases.

Furthermore, severe pain produces emotional distress (anxiety, depression, frustration), which in turn further lowers the pain threshold, and so it continues. Now we have central hypersensitivity occurring in the brain and spinal cord, in addition to visceral hypersensitivity in the bowel that leads to chronic GI pain. With central hypersensitivity, the brain-gut vicious cycle of chronic pain can produce chronic pain even when there is minimal or no injury in the gut. But there is more....

### *Neuroplasticity*

While in medical school in the 1960s, I was taught that brain cells don't grow after birth; they just die out as would occur with a stroke or a brain disease like Alzheimer's. We now know, however, that even the adult brain is neuroplastic. In other words, brain cells can shrink and grow. Chronic and severe stress, post-traumatic stress disorder (PTSD) from early trauma, or chronic pain can cause deterioration of brain cells, what we call "neurodegeneration." Brain imaging studies show that patients with chronic GI pain or severe stress have fewer cells in their pain control area than people without pain. Conversely, increased physical or mental activity increases nerve cell growth (i.e., neurogenesis). Importantly, brain cell growth can lead to lasting clinical improvement when using treatments for DGBI, such as central neuromodulators and behavioral therapy.

For more than 10 years, Johannah Ruddy experienced chronic and severe abdominal pain from post-infection IBS that began after acute gastroenteritis.[30] It was made worse by high levels of stress and PTSD from childhood abuse and trauma, causing the pain to worsen over time as the pain provided additional stress, frustration, and impaired quality of life. Now it's almost gone! For Johannah, the proper use of medications, increased knowledge to self-manage the disorder, and the benefits of an optimized patient-provider relationship (see Part 3) made this happen.[30, 31] Hear her personal account at **https://romedross.video/JohannahStory**. Johannah's story exemplifies our newer understanding of how chronic GI illness can rewire the brain-gut axis and how proper treatment can reverse this process.

### *What Doctors Need to Do*

From a clinical perspective, doctors need to discern when a patient's pain is coming primarily from the gut or the brain, or both so that they can optimize the clinical interaction and the treatment plan. When pain is intermittent and relates to eating or defecation, the pain is caused primarily by increased nerve signals arising from the gut, and treatment targets the bowel. Conversely, when pain is chronic and severe, does not change with bowel function or bodily activities, and is associated with emotional distress, the brain's pain control mechanisms are failing to work correctly, and we direct the treatment to improve those mechanisms.

The Rome IV classification of centrally mediated disorders refers to two diagnoses in which the brain plays a dominant role in the abdominal pain. These include Centrally Mediated Abdominal Pain Syndrome (CAPS) and a new diagnosis, Narcotic Bowel Syndrome (NBS), also called Opioid-Induced GI Hyperalgesia

## D1. Centrally Mediated Abdominal Pain Syndrome (CAPS)

CAPS is characterized by continuous, nearly continuous, or frequently recurring severe abdominal pain. It is only rarely related to gut function, and no other disease or DGBI explains these symptoms. Patients who have CAPS also suffer from impairments in many areas of their life, including work, intimacy, social activities, family functioning, and caregiving for self or others. Patients may also experience other painful symptoms and disorders, such as fibromyalgia, pelvic pain, and chronic fatigue syndrome. It's no surprise, then, that psychological features like anxiety, depression, and post-traumatic stress disorder often co-occur. The pain tends to persist over a long time, and it dominates the patient's life. Unfortunately, patients are susceptible to experiencing multiple, often unnecessary procedures in seeking other diagnoses as well as surgical interventions to treat the pain complaints. However, these tests come back negative, and surgical treatments for "adhesions," gallbladder dysfunction, or "chronic diverticulitis" are misdirected because they are incorrectly attributed to being the cause of the pain when that is rarely the case. Ms. Byers' case discussed in the introduction represents this diagnosis.

***Pathophysiology.*** We have just discussed the physiological basis for CAPS. Brain imaging studies of patients with chronic GI pain show abnormalities in the functioning of pain control areas of the brain and fewer numbers of brain cells. Figure 14 shows reduced brain cell density in patients with chronic GI pain.

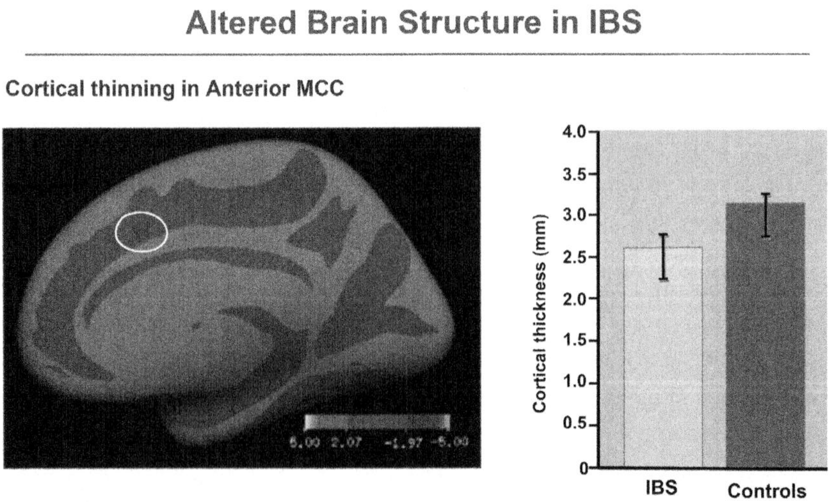


Figure 14. How chronic GI pain affects brain cell density. This image demonstrates brain cell density in patients with chronic GI pain (IBS) when compared to healthy subjects. The red area in the brain image shows that the anterior mid-cingulate cortex, the area that controls GI pain, is thinner than normal. Note too, how the amount of thinning of GI pain (yellow bar) compared to controls (blue bar). From Blankstein U et al. Altered brain structure in irritable bowel syndrome. Potential contributions of pre-existing and disease-driven factors. Gastroenterology 2010; 138:1783–1789.

We also know that the psychological distress resulting from chronic pain amplifies the experience of pain. Patients with chronic pain commonly suffer from anxiety, depression, and PTSD. The pain experience also leads to further difficulties such as feelings of lack of control, vulnerability, loss of self-efficacy, shame, and even stigmatization. These effects lend additional rationale for the use of psychological treatments to re-establish the patient's control in managing their CAPS. They also indicate how much more work is needed to educate the medical community on the legitimacy of this disorder and the effectiveness of modern treatments.

***Clinical Evaluation.***

**Rome IV Criteria for Centrally Mediated Abdominal Pain Syndrome (D1)**

Must include all of the following:

1. Continuous or nearly continuous abdominal pain
2. No or only occasional relationship of pain with physiological events (e.g., eating, defecation, or menses)
3. Pain limits some aspect of daily functioning including work, intimacy, social or leisure activities, family life, and caregiving for self or others
4. The pain is not feigned
5. Pain is not explained by another structural or functional gastrointestinal disorder or other medical condition

In addition to these Rome IV criteria, the duration of pain is of great importance because, as previously discussed, the diagnostic approach to acute abdominal pain is entirely different from that of long-standing chronic abdominal pain. With acute abdominal pain, the doctor needs to think about bowel obstruction, ulcers, pancreatitis, inflammatory bowel disease, diverticulitis, and gall bladder disease, for example. These disorders are relatively short-lived, and skilled doctors find them relatively easy to diagnose. Conversely, when pain is chronic, and the initial studies, as discussed below, have been done, there are relatively few diagnostic options to consider. Chronic pain ***is*** the diagnosis.

The diagnostic evaluation consists of a clinical and psychosocial assessment, observation of symptom-reporting behaviors, a physical examination, and, in the absence of alarm features, conservative and cost-effective efforts to exclude other medical disorders.

A careful medical history includes obtaining the description of the pain, its impact, and its consequences. The pain in CAPS is constant, nearly constant, or frequently recurring, pretty much every day, and is associated with loss of daily functioning, which is often quite severe. The pain is not or is only occasionally associated with bowel movements, eating, or menses. The abdominal location is different from chronic pelvic pain, though these conditions may co-occur much like other chronic pain conditions, and there is often a continuum of painful experiences beginning in childhood or recurring over time. The overlap with other painful disorders demonstrates the brain's inability to control the nerve signals coming from various parts of the body.

A history of loss (e.g., death of a parent, hysterectomy), early trauma, or abuse are common occurrences in patients with CAPS. My research has shown that their presence does not cause CAPS. Instead, emotional distress can worsen the severity of the pain and reduce coping capability.[32, 33] By asking a few questions, the doctor can appraise the clinical features of CAPS, identify key psychosocial contributions to the disorder, and increase confidence in the diagnosis.

When patients meet the Rome IV diagnostic criteria for CAPS and have a long-standing history of pain, no alarm features, and no other diagnostic findings, a diagnosis of CAPS is assumed. Now, the doctor must shift from further testing to focus on treatment. Sometimes, the evaluation may reveal other medical findings (e.g., renal cysts or gallstones). A discerning doctor will understand that these findings are frequently unrelated to the pain and communicate that to the patient.

***Treatment.*** Management of CAPS relies on establishing a productive patient-doctor relationship and offering management that encompasses a combination of pharmacological and psychological treatment options. Patients must enter into a therapeutic relationship, with shared responsibility and with a focus on moving away from evaluation and cure toward adaptation to chronic symptoms. Doctors need to accept CAPS as a real disorder, offer empathy, validate the patients' feelings, set realistic treatment goals, educate and reassure the patient about the nature of their condition, and provide treatment choices rather than directives.

The severity of the pain and the degree of disability will help to determine the best treatment. Central neuromodulators that improve pain are the basis for treatment. These may include tricyclic antidepressants such as Elavil (amitriptyline) or Norpramin (desipramine), or serotonin-norepinephrine reuptake inhibitors (SNRIs) such as Cymbalta (duloxetine) or Savella (milnacipran). Serotonin reuptake inhibitors (SSRIs) are not helpful for chronic abdominal pain. If the patient does not respond to the medication, the next step is to increase the dose or add a second central neuromodulator. My research has shown that if a single central neuromodulator is not successful, adding Seroquel (quetiapine) provides further benefit.[34] Brain-gut behavioral treatment, including cognitive-behavioral therapy (CBT) or hypnosis, can complement pharmacological treatment, and the combination may work better than either alone. The Rome Foundation has a network of mental health providers who are highly skilled in treating patients with DGBI, including CAPS (**https://romedross.video/RomeGIPsych**). When needed, a referral can be made to a multidisciplinary functional GI or pain treatment center that provides comprehensive assessment and treatment. Doctors should avoid pain centers that prescribe opioids, as that can worsen the condition (see Narcotic Bowel Syndrome below).

## D2. Narcotic Bowel Syndrome (NBS)/Opioid-Induced GI Hyperalgesia

Since I am a gastroenterologist also trained in psychiatry, other doctors frequently refer patients to me who have long-standing and severe abdominal pain and are taking high dosages of narcotics. Narcotics are either opiates—naturally-occurring medications derived from the poppy plant (e.g., codeine or morphine)—or opioids, which are synthetically produced medications, such as Percocet (oxycodone) or Dilaudid (hydromorphone). Over the years, I noticed that a large proportion of these patients were taking very high doses of narcotics. Even more than that, the more narcotics they were prescribed, the more intense their pain became. How could this be? About 15 years ago, I published a series of patients who I described to have Narcotic Bowel Syndrome (NBS).[35] When given narcotics, these patients paradoxically "upregulate" their pain receptors, so the pain increases. If that is true, what would happen if you took them off the narcotics? The idea of detoxifying patients with such severe pain was a scary proposition at the time; what if they got worse? I brought the patients into the hospital at the University of North Carolina and systematically took them off the narcotics. Their pain improved.[36] Figure 15 demonstrates how well these patients did in their pain scores once they were no

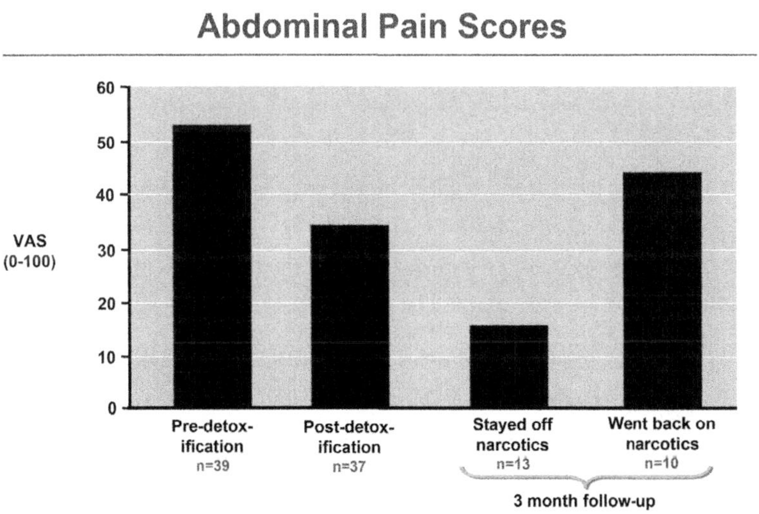


**Figure 15.** Improvement in abdominal pain after opioid detoxification in patients with Narcotic Bowel Syndrome. This graph shows the average amount of pain (from 0–100) in patients hospitalized with narcotic bowel syndrome who were detoxified from the opioids and followed for 3 months. The first bar shows that the average pain score was over 50, but after the opioids were withdrawn over about 7 days, the score dropped to about 35. If patients stayed off the narcotics for 3 months, the pain reduced further to 17. However, for those who went back on narcotics, the pain score reverted to almost pre-detoxification values. This study shows that opioids contribute to more severe pain.[36] From Drossman DA et al. Diagnosis, characterization, and 3-month outcome after detoxification of 39 patients with Narcotic Bowel Syndrome. Am J Gastroenterol. 2012;107:1426–1440.

longer taking opioids, and led to greater recognition of NBS, which became a new diagnosis for Rome IV.

By definition, we characterize NBS by the paradoxical development of or an increase in abdominal pain that occurs with continuous or increasing dosages of opioids. This disorder can occur with patients having DGBI or other chronic GI diseases like inflammatory bowel disease or chronic pancreatitis. It can also occur with patients having painful malignant or non-malignant diseases, or even in patients who receive high dosages of narcotics when recovering from surgery. As we've shown, the pain in patients with NBS will significantly improve or be entirely relieved when we withdraw the opioids.

***Pathophysiology.*** NBS seems to occur in only about 5% of patients given high-dose opioids. However, it is essential to identify these individuals so they can be treated appropriately by detoxification. The most favored reason NBS occurs is that specific cells in the spinal cord and brain, called glial cells, seem to become inflamed or activated when exposed to opioids. This causes a chemical response that sensitizes the nerves and produces central hypersensitivity. We call this Opioid-Induced Central Hyperalgesia, another name for NBS.

***Clinical Evaluation.***

**Rome IV Criteria for Narcotic Bowel Syndrome/Opioid-Induced GI Hyperalgesia (NBS) (D2)**

Must include all of the following:

1. Chronic or frequently recurring abdominal pain that is treated with acute high-dose or chronic narcotics
2. The nature and intensity of the pain is not explained by a current or previous GI diagnosis
3. Must include two or more of the following:
    a. The pain worsens or incompletely resolves with continued or escalating dosages of narcotics
    b. There is marked worsening of pain when the narcotic dose wanes and improvement when narcotics are re-instituted (soar and crash)
    c. There is a progression of the frequency, duration, and intensity of pain episodes

Pain must occur most days.

A patient may have a structural diagnosis (e.g., inflammatory bowel disease, chronic pancreatitis), but the character or activity of the disease process is not sufficient to explain the pain.

Importantly, the pain in NBS is out of proportion to the severity of the disorder and may occur when there is no other disease. When the doctor prescribes the narcotics even for appropriate reasons, the fact that they cause increasing pain is the keynote diagnostic feature and, unfortunately, is not always recognized. Eventually, the abdominal pain becomes constant and severe in the face of ongoing opioid treatment and may be associated with Opioid-Induced Constipation (OIC, previously discussed). These patients suffer greatly and commonly have anxiety and depression. They may have had extensive laboratory studies, which are usually normal. The combination of being on narcotics, meeting the Rome IV criteria, and having these negative studies is enough to make a diagnosis of NBS.

***Treatment.*** Many patients with NBS might not see going off narcotics as a logical option. They often believe these are the only medications that have helped them, and they fear being abandoned with worsening pain. They also feel stigmatized by others, whom they perceive as judging them for "drug-seeking" or having a psychiatric problem. An optimal patient-doctor relationship, achieved through trust and excellent communication, is a prerequisite for successful treatment. The doctor must commit to work with the patient and discuss the nature of NBS and options for treatment, including opiate detoxification. Mutual trust and a shared plan of care are facilitated through empathy, acceptance, and validation of the reality of the pain and its impact on the patient's life. The doctor must also clarify that the pain will get better with proper treatment. Treatment entails gradual removal of the narcotics usually over several days by IV withdrawal, and the use of central neuromodulators to raise the patient's pain threshold and treat concurrent psychological distress if it is present.[36] Friends and family members are enlisted to discuss the goals of the treatment, to ensure their support during the process, and to help prevent relapse after stopping the narcotics. Ancillary providers (e.g., psychologists or psychiatrists, the primary care doctor, and the doctor assistant) can help with the care. Most importantly, the doctor needs to reaffirm a willingness to continue with the patient, regardless of the outcome.

## E. Gallbladder and Sphincter of Oddi (SO) Disorders[20]

"I'm having a gallbladder attack!" To understand what this means, we first need to learn about the structure and function of the gallbladder and bile duct. The gallbladder is a bag-like receptacle or reservoir for the bile produced by the liver. The bile goes through the hepatic and cystic ducts into the gallbladder, where it stays until there is a meal. With a meal, the gallbladder contracts and sends the bile into the duodenum through the cystic duct, the common bile duct and the Sphincter of Oddi. Once the bile enters the duodenum and intestines, it helps to break down fat to allow its digestion and absorption into the body (see Figure 16).

Sometimes the gallbladder produces gallstones (cholelithiasis), usually made of cholesterol but occasionally are pigment stones. Most often, gallstones don't produce symptoms; the gallstones just sit in the gallbladder. However, if the gallbladder contracts and pushes a stone out, it may get stuck in the narrow portion of the cystic duct. Pressure backs up and stretches the cystic duct and gallbladder, causing

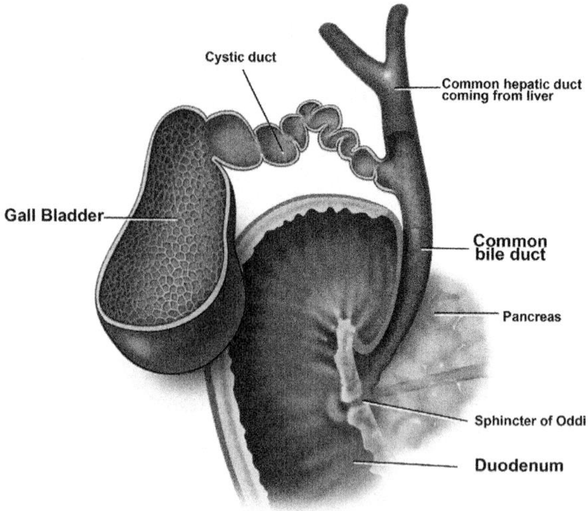


**Figure 16.** The anatomy of the gallbladder and biliary system. Bile made in the liver enters through the hepatic ducts, the common bile duct, the cystic duct, and then into the gallbladder. After a meal, the gallbladder contracts sending the bile through the cystic duct, the common bile duct, and the Sphincter of Oddi into the duodenum to digest and absorb the fat.

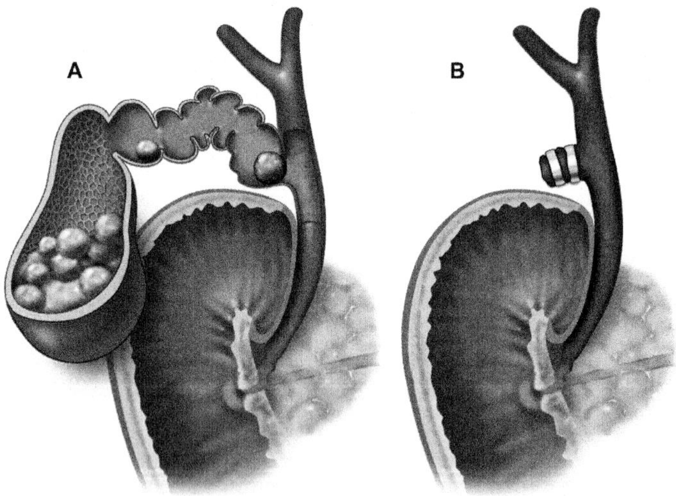


**Figure 17.** Gallbladder with stones and after removing the gallbladder. Figure 17A shows a gallbladder with gallstones (cholelithiasis). A gallstone is obstructing the cystic duct, leading to a gallbladder attack (cholecystitis) with biliary colic. Cholecystectomy (removing the gallbladder along with the gallstones) is the treatment of choice. Figure 17B shows the biliary system (common bile duct) after cholecystectomy. Notably, even without the gallbladder present, pressure may still build up in the bile duct from the bile accumulating if the Sphincter of Oddi does not empty the bile into the duodenum. The increased pressure in the bile duct can also cause biliary pain, which is relieved by endoscopic sphincterotomy.

the pain we call Biliary Pain. The blockage of the gallstone is what occurs with a typical gallbladder attack (Figure 17a). Surgically removing the gallbladder then is the treatment for cholelithiasis, as shown in Figure 17b.

The gallbladder and Sphincter of Oddi disorders are the main DGBI where the patient can get biliary pain but has no evidence for structural causes such as gallstones, tumors, strictures, and other kinds of blockages. These disorders occur either with poor emptying of the gallbladder (Functional Gallbladder Disorder), or if the gallbladder is absent, from an inability of the Sphincter of Oddi to relax appropriately to let the bile enter into the duodenum. Removal of the gallbladder or endoscopically opening the blocked sphincter are the treatments for these disorders. For further information go to: **https://romedross.video/Q_A_BilliaryPain**.

## E1. Biliary Pain

Biliary Pain, also called Biliary Colic, is intense, episodic pain in the upper right quadrant of the abdomen under the rib cage. It can last for hours at a time and is often so severe that it is associated with nausea and vomiting and usually brings the patient to the emergency room.

***Pathophysiology.*** The pain occurs due to increased pressure within the gallbladder or bile duct. Increased pressure leads to stretching of the gallbladder or bile duct, causing pain (colic).

***Clinical Evaluation.*** As discussed below, the doctor needs to be sure there is no blockage due to gallstones, tumors, or stricture.

**Rome IV Criteria for Biliary Pain (E1)**

Pain located in the epigastrium and/or right upper quadrant and all of the following:

1. Builds up to a steady level and lasting 30 minutes or longer
2. Occurring at different intervals (not daily)
3. Severe enough to interrupt daily activities or lead to an emergency department visit
4. Not significantly (<20%) related to bowel movements
5. Not significantly (<20%) relieved by postural change or acid suppression

*Supportive criteria:*

The pain may be associated with:

1. Nausea and vomiting
2. Radiation to the back and/or right infrasubscapular region
3. Waking from sleep

***Treatment.*** Treatment depends on the cause of Biliary Pain.

## E1a. Functional Gallbladder Disorder (FGBD)

Functional Gallbladder Disorder (FGBD) occurs when the patient meets Rome IV criteria for Biliary Pain, and the gallbladder is present, but there are no gallstones or sediment (sludge). Testing to exclude other causes is most often done by abdominal or endoscopic ultrasound (EUS), which are accurate methods to identify these other causes of Biliary Colic.

***Pathophysiology.*** FGBD is believed to be due to incomplete emptying of the gallbladder. The scintigraphic test to evaluate slow gallbladder emptying (CCK-CS) involves the intravenous administration of technetium 99m (Tc 99m), which is excreted into the biliary tract and concentrated in the gallbladder. The rate at which the Tc 99m empties from the gallbladder is called the ejection fraction (EF). If the EF is low (usually 40% or less), this diagnosis is supported. FGBD is thought to be a motility disorder, but the slow emptying may also cause secondary inflammation of the gallbladder. On occasion, a delayed EF may be due to tiny gallstones (microlithiasis) that are difficult to detect.

***Clinical Evaluation.***

**Rome IV Criteria for Functional Gallbladder Disorder (E1a)**

Must include both of the following:

1. Criteria for Biliary Pain
2. Absence of gallstones or other structural pathology

*Supportive criteria:*

1. Low ejection fraction on gallbladder scintigraphy
2. Normal liver enzymes, conjugated bilirubin, and amylase/lipase

Once the Rome IV diagnostic criteria are fulfilled and no gallstones are found (based on abdominal ultrasound, or if needed, endoscopic ultrasound), a diagnosis of FGBD is made. However, other tests, like upper endoscopy, CT scan, or MRI, may be required to rule out peptic ulcer disease, other intestinal diseases, or pancreatitis. Often, if the pains are typical and severe and no gallstones are found, the diagnosis of FGBD is made without further studies

***Treatment.*** Symptoms suggestive of FGBD often resolve on their own. Because Biliary Colic may be a frightening experience, the doctor needs to provide education and reassurance. Antispasmodics such as Levsin (hyoscyamine) or Bentyl (dicyclomine) are often prescribed for mild episodes. When the episodes are more severe or frequent, I prescribe central neuromodulators such as TCAs, including Elavil (amitriptyline), Norpramin (desipramine), or SNRIs like Cymbalta (duloxetine) to prevent or reduce the frequency of episodes. Surgical removal of the gallbladder (cholecystectomy) is done when these methods fail, and the likelihood of its benefit increases when the ejection fraction is <40%. Unfortunately, the surgical results vary, and I see a high number of patients that continue with Biliary Pain after a cholecystectomy (post-cholecystectomy pain). For these reasons, I frequently rely on medical treatments.

## E1b. Functional Biliary Sphincter of Oddi (SO) Disorder

Figure 17b shows the biliary system after cholecystectomy. As discussed, Biliary Pain (see E1) can also occur after the gallbladder is removed because there is no gallbladder reservoir to hold the bile. Pressure builds up as bile accumulates in the common bile duct when the Sphincter of Oddi does not relax properly to empty the bile.

***Pathophysiology.*** When the Sphincter of Oddi does not relax enough to release the bile into the duodenum, pressure in the bile duct increases, and this produces the biliary pain. Recent research indicates that this may not be the full picture. The blockage may also cause bile duct inflammation, leading to visceral hypersensitivity (see previous discussions). In most patients, reducing the pressure in the bile duct, by cutting the Sphincter of Oddi (endoscopic sphincterotomy), can prevent future pressure increases and pain episodes. However, some patients continue to have pain episodes even after sphincterotomy, and this may be due to visceral hypersensitivity. Hypersensitivity may also include other areas of the biliary tract, and even the duodenum.

***Clinical Evaluation.***

**Rome IV Criteria for Functional Biliary Sphincter of Oddi Disorder (E1b)**

Must include all of the following:

1. Criteria for biliary pain
2. Elevated liver enzymes or dilated bile duct, but not both
3. Absence of bile duct stones or other structural abnormalities

*Supportive criteria:*

1. Normal amylase/lipase
2. Abnormal sphincter of Oddi manometry
3. Abnormal hepatobiliary scintigraphy

Once the Rome IV diagnostic criteria are fulfilled and no gallstones or obstructing lesions are found (based on abdominal or endoscopic ultrasound), a diagnosis of Functional Biliary Sphincter of Oddi Disorder can be made. Other tests like a CT scan or MRI may on occasion be needed.

***Treatment.*** If symptoms are not severe, the doctor may use medical treatments. As noted for FGBD, antispasmodic medications or central neuromodulators may offer benefits. However, the standard of treatment when symptoms are moderate or severe is endoscopic sphincterotomy. Sphincterotomy involves placing the endoscope through the stomach into the duodenum. When the endoscope reaches the Sphincter of Oddi, a wire is advanced into the sphincter and the bile duct. Then the sphincter is cut by electrical cautery, and this relieves the increased pressure. The main complications, usually in inexperienced hands, would be pancreatitis, bleeding, or perforation of the duodenum or bile duct.

## F. Anorectal Disorders[21]

Everyone has experienced anorectal difficulties, but few people feel comfortable discussing them, even with their doctors. Nevertheless, we must appreciate this remarkably coordinated, muscular system that allows us to function in society. What would it be like if, like birds, we had no mechanism for continence? How valuable is it to have an anal sphincter that can differentiate solid, liquid, and gas (well, most of the time)? How much fun is it to provide such rich comedic material for entertainers? When the anorectal muscles don't work correctly, however, we experience difficulties that must be understood and treated. The anorectal disorders described here are a group of DGBI that relate primarily to problems in pelvic floor muscle functioning. When they are too weak, they produce fecal incontinence. When they contract too much, they produce rectal pain (either Levator Ani Syndrome or Proctalgia Fugax). When they are not well-coordinated, they produce Dyssynergic Defecation. Unlike many of the DGBI, diagnosis of anorectal disorders usually requires physiological testing, and treatment involves retraining the muscles, either with exercises or biofeedback.

To begin, let's understand the anatomy and functioning of the pelvic floor (Figure 18). The pelvic floor is a relatively small area of the body that, in women, is studied and treated by three medical specialties: gastroenterology, gynecology, and urology. Unfortunately, patients must sometimes go to different specialists for the same problem and may be treated differently. I find it notable, like the story of the blind men and the elephant, that each specialist understands the pelvic floor in different ways, based on their training. Medically speaking, this is simply because of the way that medical specialties have evolved since these anatomic areas and their functioning are highly coordinated. See more on pelvic floor difficulties: **https://romedross.video/QA1_24_20PFD**.

The left side of Figure 18 demonstrates that the rectum is located behind or posterior to the uterus and vagina. The vagina, in turn, is behind the urethra and bladder. These organs are held in place by a sling of pelvic floor muscles, which include the puborectalis (or levator muscle). This sling runs from the pubis, in the front or anteriorly, to the back of the rectum. Then it continues and ends just in front of the coccyx. Continence occurs because the internal and external sphincters stay contracted. Note also that the rectum is tethered by the puborectalis to form a right angle. This angle acts as a barrier to prevent stool from descending into and out of the anus. As shown on the righthand side of Figure 18, the levator muscle relaxes with defecation, thereby straightening the rectum and making it easier for

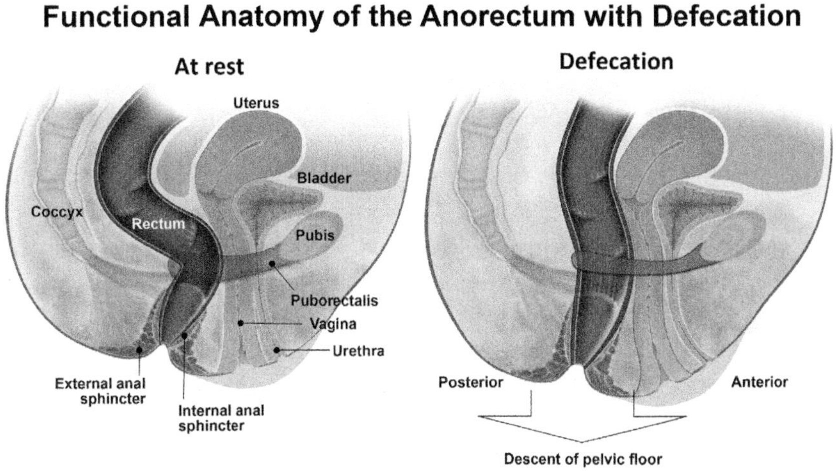


**Figure 18.** Anatomy of the pelvic floor in the female at rest and during defecation. See text above for details.

stool to descend to the anus. The sphincters also relax to ease the passage of stool, leading to the evacuation. Now we can discuss the anorectal disorders that occur when anorectal functioning is impaired.

## F1. Fecal Incontinence (FI)

Fecal incontinence is defined by the recurrent uncontrolled passage of fecal material for at least 3 months. While fecal staining of the underwear may relate to poor hygiene, prolapsing hemorrhoids, or rectal prolapse, FI is usually due to failure of the muscles to function correctly, leading to difficulty maintaining continence. FI can be made worse by any condition that causes diarrhea, and if present, diarrhea also needs to be treated. Multiple vaginal deliveries, advanced age, smoking, gynecological surgical procedures, or other injuries to the anal sphincter, obesity, and other diseases like diabetes are likely to cause FI or to worsen it.

Persons with FI suffer emotionally from this disorder, perhaps more so than with most of the DGBI. Poor bowel control restricts social life. Patients need to determine toilet location, be concerned about hygiene and odor issues, and avoid physical activities. They experience fear and embarrassment due to the unpredictability of their bowel habits. Co-existent psychological problems may include anxiety and depression, poor self-esteem, and problems with sexual relationships.

***Pathophysiology.*** Anal sphincter weakness is the most frequently identified abnormality in FI. Among older women, approximately 40% have reduced sphincter pressure during rest, and 80% have reduced sphincter pressure during squeezing. Internal anal sphincter dysfunction occurs after obstetric injury or from thinning of the sphincter due to advanced age or other diseases. Internal and external sphincter function is best determined by anorectal ultrasound.

***Clinical Evaluation.***

> **Rome IV Criteria for Fecal Incontinence (F1)**
>
> 1. Recurrent uncontrolled passage of fecal material in an individual with a developmental age of at least 4 years

Given the emotional impact of FI, doctors need to develop a good relationship with patients to permit discussion of the severity and nature of the symptoms and their emotional and behavioral consequences. It is vital to determine the symptoms (pain, straining), stooling pattern (frequency, amount), and their appearance (solid, liquid, or gas), as well as the degree of incontinence: staining, seepage, soiling (of underwear or bedding), and overt full incontinence. The interview should also include the impact of these symptoms on emotional state, interpersonal relationships, and daily activities. Patients with urge incontinence sense the need to defecate but cannot reach the toilet in time, while patients with passive incontinence are not aware of the presence of stool until it's too late. In general, the passage of solid stool suggests a more severe sphincter weakness than liquid stool alone. FI can be made worse by laxatives, artificial sweeteners, or a history of anorectal surgical procedures. Conversely, agents that create constipation may predispose to the retention of stool and overflow diarrhea. Here, liquid stool passes over the retained stool and leaks out.

The physical examination includes an abdominal and rectal examination. Inspection of the anus may show scars from previous surgery or obstetric injury or the presence of inflammation or fecal soiling. The doctor also tests for the "anal wink," where stroking of the anal area causes a reflex that contracts the sphincter. When not present, this may suggest a neurological disease. Then the doctor inserts the finger into the rectum to test the degree of tension of the sphincter and levator muscles, both at rest and after squeezing. An anorectal motility study can more thoroughly test the strength and function of the pelvic floor muscles. In this study, a balloon is inserted into the rectum. Then the patient squeezes and relaxes the pelvic floor muscle while pressures are recorded and displayed on the computer.

***Treatment.*** Management of FI must address all factors that contribute to it. Lactose or fructose restriction may help if the patient is intolerant of these sugars. Psyllium fiber (e.g., Metamucil) can help to firm up the stool. Loperamide (Imodium), 2 mg, given before meals or after a loose bowel movement, can improve stool consistency and increase the internal sphincter tone. Lomotil (diphenoxylate and atropine) is an alternative to loperamide but may produce more side effects. A tricyclic antidepressant, like Elavil (amitriptyline), can also improve FI in some patients. When constipation is severe, there may be fecal impaction and overflow incontinence. This requires treatment to empty the rectum, which is done by using a Golytely or Miralax (PEG solution) flush. If patients do not improve with these bowel treatments, periodic rectal cleansing is a practical solution.

Behavioral treatments include pelvic floor and sphincter tightening (e.g., "Kegel") exercises, which can be done by physical therapists or by self-learning. I strongly recommend anorectal biofeedback therapy because of its high success rate; it shows an even more significant benefit than Kegel exercises.[37]

When FI becomes more severe, surgical anal sphincter repair is often considered but is not useful for everyone long term. The US Food and Drug Administration has approved two treatments for FI: stimulation of the sacral nerve and injection of a specific bulking agent—dextranomer in hyaluronic acid (NASHA Dx)—underneath the mucous lining of the anus. When these treatments are being considered, I recommend consultations with gastroenterologists and colorectal surgeons to determine their possible value.

## F2. Functional Anorectal Pain

The functional anorectal pain disorders indeed are "*pains in the arse.*" They are identified based on the duration of pain and the presence or absence of anorectal tenderness on rectal examination. These syndromes often overlap in their clinical presentation.

### F2a. Levator Ani Syndrome

Levator Ani Syndrome is attributed to tension in this muscle producing pain often described as a vague, dull ache, or a sensation of pressure high in the rectum lasting 30 minutes or longer. It is often worse when sitting than when standing or lying down. Physical examination reveals tenderness when the doctor presses on the pelvic floor (posterior traction of the levator) muscle. Other structural disorders of the pelvic floor must be excluded.

***Pathophysiology.*** Levator Ani Syndrome is thought to result from spasm of pelvic floor muscles and elevated anal resting pressures. Perhaps it's no surprise that a large number of patients with this syndrome also have Dyssynergic Defecation (see F3a). This suggests that rectoanal incoordination may be a pathophysiological explanation for Levator Ani Syndrome.

***Clinical Evaluation.***

**Rome IV Criteria for Levator Ani Syndrome (F2a)**

Must include all of the following:

1. Chronic or recurrent rectal pain or aching
2. Episodes last 30 minutes or longer
3. Tenderness during traction on the puborectalis
4. Exclusion of other causes of rectal pain, such as inflammatory bowel disease, intramuscular abscess and fissure, thrombosed hemorrhoids, prostatitis, coccygodynia, and major structural alterations of the pelvic floor

Diagnosis is based primarily on the presence of characteristic symptoms and physical examination findings, as noted in the criteria above—i.e., rectal pain lasting 30 minutes or longer and tenderness upon traction of the puborectalis. Evaluation often includes sigmoidoscopy, ultrasound, and pelvic imaging to exclude other possible diseases.

***Treatment.*** Treatments can include muscle relaxant medications such as Valium (diazepam) and Flexeril (cyclobenzaprine), digital massage of the levator ani muscles to relax them, electrogalvanic stimulation, and Sitz baths. However, much like the treatment of FI, I recommend anorectal biofeedback because it is more successful than digital massage or electrogalvanic stimulation.[38]

## F2b. Unspecified Functional Anorectal Pain

With this diagnosis, the patient has the same symptoms as Levator Ani Syndrome. However, there is no tenderness when the doctor presses on the levator muscle during the rectal exam.

**Rome IV Criteria for Unspecified Functional Anorectal Pain (F2b)**
Symptom criteria for chronic Levator Ani Syndrome but no tenderness during posterior traction on the puborectalis muscle

***Treatment.*** Treatment is the same as for Levator Ani Syndrome (F2a).

## F2c. Proctalgia Fugax

This disorder relates to recurrent episodes of pain in the rectal area, lasting for a few seconds to several minutes (but no more than 30 minutes) and then completely disappearing. The pain has been described as cramping, gnawing, aching, or stabbing; and may range from uncomfortable to unbearable. An attack may interrupt normal activities, and symptoms may awaken the patient from sleep. Interestingly, patients don't usually go to the doctor with this complaint because the symptoms are so fleeting that the diagnosis is only made when the doctor queries about these characteristic symptoms. Perhaps this is why, in the mid-20th century, male medical students were the first to self-identify and report the disorder (there were very few female students then). They were considered stressed, perfectionistic, anxious, and hypochondriacal. We now know, however, that Proctalgia Fugax occurs in males and females, and while it may be precipitated by stress, it is not necessarily related to psychiatric disturbances.

***Pathophysiology.*** The short duration and sporadic, infrequent nature of this disorder makes it difficult to understand the cause, but abnormal muscle contractions may be responsible for the pain. Attacks of Proctalgia Fugax may be caused by stressful life events or anxiety.

***Clinical Evaluation.***

**Rome IV Criteria for Proctalgia Fugax (F2c)**

Must include all of the following:

1. Recurrent episodes of pain localized to the rectum and unrelated to defecation
2. Episodes last from seconds to minutes, with a maximum duration of 30 minutes
3. There is no anorectal pain between episodes
4. Exclusion of other causes of rectal pain, such as inflammatory bowel disease, intramuscular abscess and fissure, thrombosed hemorrhoids, prostatitis, coccygodynia, and major structural alterations of the pelvic floor

Diagnosis is based on the presence of characteristic symptoms as above and the exclusion of other anorectal and pelvic diagnoses.

***Treatment.*** For most patients, episodes are so brief that treatment is impractical and so sporadic that prevention is not feasible. Because it is harmless, treatment must first include reassurance and explanation. However, patients with frequent symptoms may be treated with antispasmodic or nitroglycerine pills or ointment to relax the muscles.

## F3. Functional Defecation Disorders (FDD)

Patients with these disorders have difficulty evacuating due to poor coordination of their pelvic floor muscles. In Figure 18, note that the puborectalis muscle relaxes with defecation, thereby straightening the rectal angle, which permits easier passage of stool. With FDD, this does not occur. Instead, when the person tries to defecate, the puborectalis muscle either contracts excessively or fails to relax sufficiently. The rectal appearance, therefore, stays as in the left side of Figure 18, and the rectal angle acts as a barrier to stool passage. In some cases, inadequate ability to propel the stool, meaning that there is a reduction of propulsive forces, may also impede defecation.

So, the symptoms of FDD relate to excessive straining and a feeling of incomplete evacuation, which may lead some patients to use their fingers to help remove (disimpact) the stool. However, these symptoms are not sufficient to make a diagnosis of FDD because other disorders can also lead to difficulty evacuating (see the Clinical Evaluation, below). That is why the criteria for FDDs must rely on both symptoms and physiological testing.

***Pathophysiology.*** Patients with FDD likely have an acquired behavioral disorder; in other words, they have become conditioned not to relax the pelvic floor correctly. Why might this occur? Many of my patients report that these symptoms began in childhood, which is when the child first learns to use these muscles for defecating or for withholding stool. So, for example, if toilet training is positively reinforced, defecation becomes easy. However, certain factors may interfere with this process. Many patients recall feeling uncomfortable in grade school when they had to use toilets outside the home, so they "held back." In this way, they may have conditioned themselves not to relax the pelvic floor when they needed to "go" in other places. Similarly, many people find it difficult to evacuate when traveling and using local toilet facilities, and they become constipated. Furthermore, a high proportion of patients with FDD have a childhood history of sexual abuse, and this also contributes to the inability to relax the pelvic floor because of anxiety and psychological stress that increases pelvic floor muscle tension. But the good news is that just as the muscles have become conditioned not to relax, they can be re-trained to relax appropriately. That is the basis for treating FDD by using pelvic floor exercises and biofeedback, with excellent success.

***Clinical Evaluation.***

**Rome IV Criteria for Functional Defecation Disorders (FDD) (F3)**

Must include all of the following:

1. The patient must satisfy diagnostic criteria for functional constipation and/or irritable bowel syndrome with constipation
2. During repeated attempts to defecate, there must be features of impaired evacuation, as demonstrated by two of the following three tests:
   a. Abnormal balloon expulsion test
   b. Abnormal anorectal evacuation pattern with manometry or anal surface EMG
   c. Impaired rectal evacuation by imaging

*Subcategories F3a and F3b apply to patients who satisfy criteria for FDD (F3)*

FDD is sub-categorized as follows.

**F3a. Diagnostic Criteria for Inadequate Defecatory Propulsion** – In this disorder, the patient does not push down very well when defecating, so there is an insufficient force to push out the stool—a condition that is measured using anorectal manometry. This can also occur with inappropriate contraction of the anal sphincter or pelvic floor muscles. Inadequate propulsion is measured using anorectal manometry.

**Rome IV Criteria for Inadequate Defecatory Propulsion (F3a)**

1. Must first satisfy Rome IV criteria for FDD (F3)
2. Inadequate propulsive forces as measured with manometry with or without inappropriate contraction of the anal sphincter and/or pelvic floor muscles

**F3b. Diagnostic Criteria for Dyssynergic Defecation** – Dyssynergic Defecation is the more common FDD. Here, there is an inappropriate contraction of the pelvic floor as measured by EMG or anorectal manometry, even though there are adequate propulsive forces. For more on dyssynergic defecation go to: **https://romedross.video/Q_A_DysynDefecConstip**.

> **Rome IV Criteria for Dyssynergic Defecation (F3b)**
> 1. Must first satisfy Rome IV criteria for FDD (F3)
> 2. Inappropriate contraction of the pelvic floor as measured with anal surface EMG or manometry with adequate propulsive forces during attempted defecation
>
> These criteria are defined by age- and sex-appropriate normal values for the technique.

The diagnosis of FDD is made by two or three of the symptom criteria for Functional Constipation (see Functional Constipation): prolonged excessive straining, a feeling of incomplete evacuation, and manual maneuvers to help evacuate the stool. A rectal examination is an accurate way to determine if the puborectalis doesn't correctly relax. As I have mentioned, other conditions may produce these symptoms. One of these is a rectocele, a weakening of the wall between the rectum and vagina. It can develop from repeated straining, which generates increased abdominal pressure, which then pushes the rectal wall into the vaginal area. A rectocele can also occur from multiple vaginal deliveries or surgeries that weaken this wall. A rectal and vaginal examination can make this diagnosis. When present, a rectocele can be treated by splinting (see below) or surgical repair. Other pelvic floor disorders that may produce difficulty with defecation include an enterocele (in which the intestinal contents push into the pelvic floor), or prolapse of the rectum or pelvic floor, where these structures push into and block the anal canal. All of these are due to laxity, i.e., excess relaxation of the pelvic floor structures. These diagnoses are also identified by pelvic examination and confirmed by physiological testing.

If none of these other possibilities is present, several tests can be considered to confirm the diagnosis of FDD:

- ***Balloon expulsion test.*** A deflated balloon is placed into the rectum and then inflated to about 50 ml (about 2 ounces of fluid) to simulate a stool. While sitting privately on a commode chair, the patient is asked to expel the balloon within 2 minutes. If this does not occur, the test is considered abnormal.
- ***Anorectal manometric assessment (ARM).*** This test measures the anal and rectal pressures and EMG (electromyogram) electrical activity during attempted defecation. When these tests are normal, increased pressure inside the rectum is associated with anal relaxation. A study with abnormal results will demonstrate inappropriately increased pressures or inadequate relaxation of the rectum or the anal sphincter during simulated defecation.

- ***Defecography.*** This x-ray or MRI technique provides a more detailed evaluation of the rectum and pelvic floor during attempted defecation. This test can detect structural abnormalities—for example, rectocele, enterocele, or rectal prolapse, and assess the functioning of the pelvic floor (e.g., anorectal angle at rest and during straining, a descent of the pelvic floor and the degree of rectal emptying). These abnormalities, when found, can be appropriately treated.

***Treatment.*** Numerous research studies have shown that anorectal biofeedback is a safe and effective treatment for FDD. In this treatment, pressure sensors or EMG are placed inside the anus and rectum to provide feedback to the patient on muscle activity during simulated defecation. So, for example, the patient views a computer screen that shows pressure or electrical activity. When simulating defecation, if the pressures are too high, the patient is taught how to reduce the pressures, and this reduction is viewed on the computer screen, which provides the needed feedback for reducing inappropriate pelvic floor muscle tension.

If biofeedback training is not available, a doctor or trained physical therapist can use behavioral modification methods. The patient is educated on what is being done incorrectly when they attempt to defecate. During the rectal examination, the patient is taught how to increase intra-abdominal pressure while relaxing the pelvic floor muscles. Physical therapists can also offer other pelvic floor exercises to help achieve proper relaxation. Handouts of exercises, like reverse Kegel methods, can be given to help the patient to practice. If a rectocele is present, the patient can be taught "splinting." With this technique, the patient uses a finger to push up and back either at the back of the vagina or in the area between the vagina and rectum. This prevents the rectocele pouch from forming during defecation, thereby permitting easier stool passage.

## PART 3

# Maximizing the Patient-Doctor Relationship (PDR)

*"My care changed when I was able to honestly share my symptoms, thoughts and feelings with my doctor and knew that he was going to listen and try to help; that made me feel validated and empowered."*
—Johannah Ruddy, MEd, Co-author

Johannah Ruddy's statement[30] goes to the heart of this book. Having described the common DGBI and the need to use the biopsychosocial model when treating patients who have DGBI like Johannah, we want to explain how the model works within the patient-doctor relationship (PDR). How does that happen? What does that look like? It looks like effective communication between patient and doctor occurring within a relationship of mutual respect. It's where doctors use their knowledge and skills to understand and effectively respond to their patient's needs and preferences for treatment.[1] It's also a shared relationship in which the patient plays an essential role in their healing process. It looks like what we call "patient-centered care." Before we explain this relationship and specify the responsibilities it entails for doctor and patient, let's review why there's a problem with the PDR in the first place and take a look at the known benefits of a good PDR.

### The Problem with the Patient-Doctor Relationship (PDR)

We began by describing how the patient-doctor relationship has suffered because of changes in the healthcare system. Doctors are required to see more patients in less time and are obliged to handle ever more administrative duties, which shifts their focus during office visits. They also often receive less reimbursement from third-party payers than they used to and increasingly turn to tests as a seemingly time-efficient way to make a diagnosis. However, tests get only to the structural or biological abnormalities, not the patient's thoughts and feelings underlying the illness. As a result of these pressures, clinic visit time has plummeted, the medical interview (in which the doctor finds out the patient's symptoms in the context of their thoughts and feelings) is drastically shortened, and the physical examination has all but disappeared from office visits (Figure 19). These changes have undermined the PDR, and resulted in a much less satisfying experience for both patient

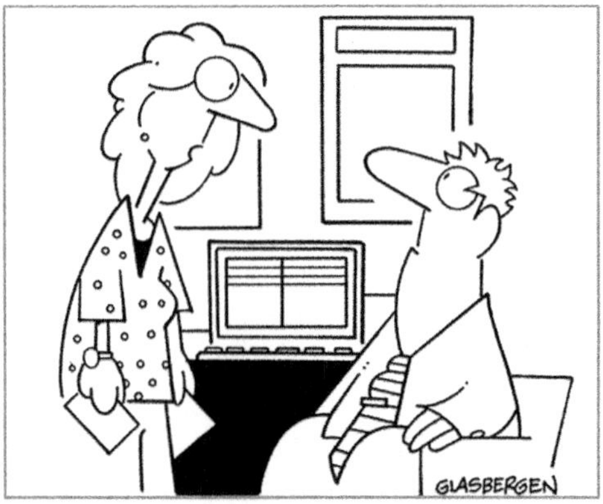


**"The doctor will be in shortly to type on the computer and update your chart. If he has time, he will ask how you're feeling and take a look at your rash."**

**Figure 19.** Changes in the healthcare system diminish the PDR

and doctor. The "art of medicine" is disappearing—and with it, much of the joy that often attended the patient-doctor partnership. Doctors have lost the connection to their patients; patients feel diminished with their role in the PDR, and often respond with frustration, and, at times, self-blame and stigmatization.[1]

The other component of this relationship failure is related, as we have stated, to the way that doctors treat patients with DGBI and other non-structurally based disorders. For these disorders, positive medical outcomes depend upon using the biopsychosocial model. However, as we have seen, Western medicine evolved based on Cartesian dualism—which conceives of the mind and body as separate—and therefore relies on the dualistic biomedical model, in which only structural abnor-

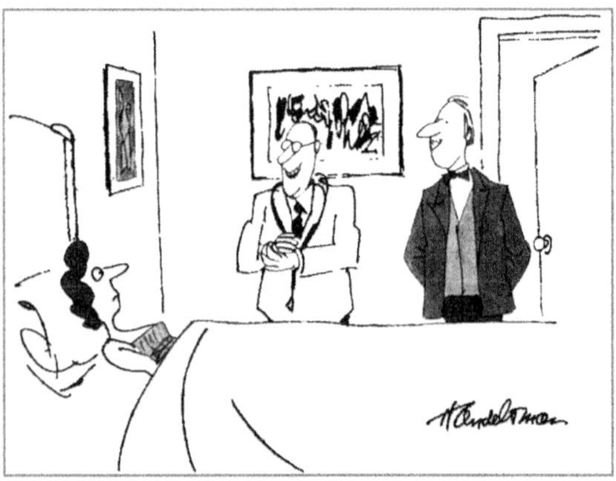

**"Well, the old body checks out. Now let's see what Doc Atkins here makes of the old mind."**

**Figure 20.** The dualistic approach in health care

malities are considered valid medical conditions. Further, the centuries-old failure to understand and appreciate the role of the biopsychosocial model as the way to understand DGBI has created a false split between patients: those with rightful suffering who have a structural disease, and those believed to have a psychiatric or even a made-up problem who have a functional illness (see Figure 20).[39]

In short, patients with functional illnesses like DGBI are often not considered medically legitimate and are treated as if they were second-class. The following video discusses the reasons for this stigmatization: **http://bit.ly/2HbpVDy**.

## Patient-Centered Care: Creating a Partnership to Optimize the PDR

Since the PDR is of primary importance in the care of patients with DGBI, communication within that relationship is essential, both for the patient's improvement and for the doctor to be able to appreciate the patient and their illness experience. However, most doctors have had little or no training in how to communicate with their patients to establish such a therapeutic relationship. Similarly, very few patients have experienced such a relationship with their doctors or imagined that they could. That is because the traditional model of care is "doctor centered." We, on the other hand, propose that the solution is through a partnership of patient-centered care. Note the differences:

*Doctor-Centered Care:*

- The doctor dominates and controls the interview
- Patient participation is limited or not expected
- Doctors are fully responsible for medical decisions
- The impact of the illness on the patient's life is not considered

*Patient-Centered Care:*

- The patient is considered the source of information
- Patient participation is active, and doctors respond to patient cues
- The evaluation is biopsychosocial and includes psychosocial factors
- Doctors use communication skills and demonstrate empathy
- Doctors provide options for treatment
- Final decisions rest with the patient

We will see the impact of patient-centered care with Johannah's story (discussed below).[30] She says, *"As a patient with a chronic GI illness and a patient advocate, I learned that when I passively accepted a doctor's directive, the outcome was nowhere as positive as it is now when I share the responsibility of care with my current provider."*

In our discussions with countless patients, their requests keep coming through: *"We are just looking for someone to listen, to care, and to provide long-term support."*

This is the lasting patient-doctor story that we all desire.[30] So now, in Part 3, we are going to present the communication skills that can fix the PDR—skills that align with patient-centered care.

## Using Communication Skills to Optimize the PDR

The movement toward patient-centered care began about 20 years ago when the Institute of Medicine (IOM) raised concerns about the presence of a "chasm" between the patient and doctor within American health care because of poor communication and doctor-centered care. The IOM sought to change this by publishing a document, "Crossing the Quality Chasm: A New Health System for the 21st Century."[40] They promoted patient-centered care as the solution, which they defined as: *"Providing care that is respectful of, and responsive to, individual patient preferences, needs and values, and ensuring that patient values guide all clinical decisions."*

They defined patient-centered care as (1) respect for your knowledge and perspective (even if it is different from the doctor's view), (2) providing physical comfort and emotional support, (3) offering education and reassurance, (4) being accessible and collaborative, and (5) making treatment decisions based on patient preferences. This approach requires you and your doctor to develop a partnership in your care and treatment.

Patient-centered care provides the basis for meaningful communication. It requires a dialog where patients and doctors communicate within the medical set-

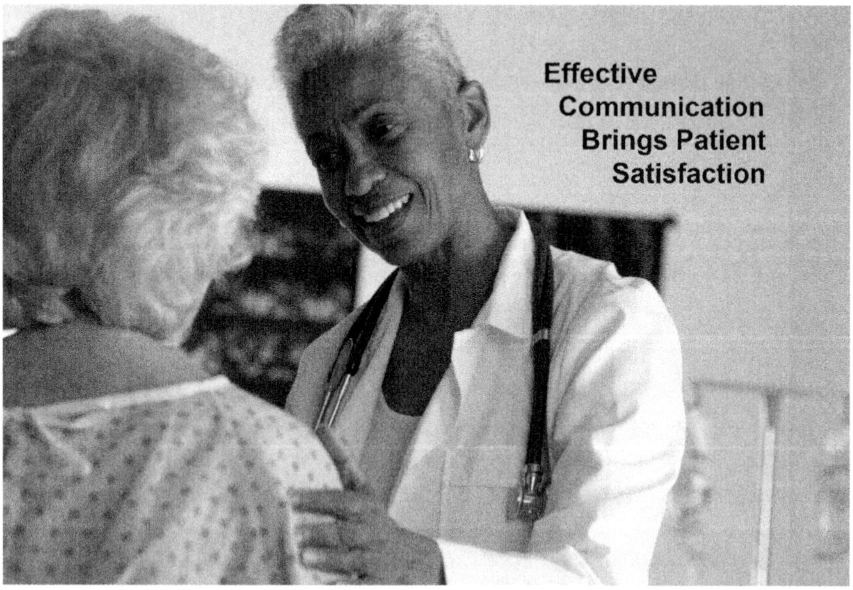


**Figure 21.** Effective communication leads to patient and doctor satisfaction

ting. Doctors learn to ask questions correctly. In turn, patients provide answers, but they need to learn how to deliver personal context and the circumstances that lead to those answers. So, learning communication skills is a two-way street.

In the sections that follow, we provide a template for you as a patient to learn what makes communication better. You can apply this information to your clinical visits and to understand your doctor's approach to you.

### *How Good Communication Skills Improve the PDR*

Implementing excellent communication skills has several benefits:[39]

1. **Improves diagnostic accuracy and clinical decisions.** When your doctor listens to you actively, addresses your agenda, empathizes with you, and validates your concerns, it encourages you to open up and give them all levels of information (clinical and psychosocial) needed for your diagnosis and managing your illness.
2. **Establishes trust.** An engaged doctor creates an environment in which you can feel safe to share deep thoughts and feelings that may be contributing to your illness. The information you give the doctor also helps them to understand how your illness impacts you, and this, in turn, facilitates shared decision making and leads to optimal treatment.
3. **Creates a collaboration of care.** With chronic illnesses such as DGBI, responsibility for improvement must involve a partnership. The use of practical communication skills and shared decision making are the foundation and hallmarks of a good PDR.
4. **Provides time efficiency.** Some doctors may believe that a patient-centered interview takes more time, but that is not correct. The doctor can construct the questions based on what you tell them—and this opens the door for you to disclose more details about your illness and your thoughts and feelings in less time. In other words, you more efficiently share your biopsychosocial world. The following video demonstrates the differences between an ineffective and effective communication style during a medical visit: **http://bit.ly/2H7MHb3**.
5. **Benefits the patient, the provider, and the clinical outcome.**[39] You benefit by getting your needs addressed, receiving clear information, and arriving at a mutual set of goals and treatment. The doctor who learns to communicate effectively also gets more satisfaction from a job well done. Finally, the clinical outcome is better because a good PDR reduces symptom severity, emotional distress, and improves the quality of life.
6. **Reduces patients' requests for additional healthcare services.** When you feel better, you stop looking for unnecessary testing to "find the answer." This lessens the burden on the healthcare system and is better for you, emotionally and financially.

Having grasped the importance and benefits of effective communication and patient-centered care, the Rome Foundation and DrossmanCare developed basic curricula to improve communication skills, including a printable study guide (**https://romedross.video/2YphMDd**) and a comprehensive program for doctors to implement these skills (**https://romedross.video/2KPTYzC**). We hope that doctors will use these communication strategies to understand the patient's symptoms fully, how they experience their illness, its impact on their life, and their needs and concerns.[1]

Before we list these strategies, let's share what Johannah has learned—as a patient with chronic GI illness—about the PDR, and illustrate the importance of communication in her long journey to wellness.[30] We also want to address some of the issues that negatively affected her care and hear how her doctor participated in her healing process.[31]

### *Johannah's Story as a Patient with a Chronic GI Illness*

*Pain is something we all experience. Growing up as the oldest of four children in a conservative, Protestant, middle-class family, I learned that you had to tolerate pain and learn to deal with it. Getting sick or injured was not an excuse for sympathy or a day off from school. It was expected that you powered through and sometimes thought of it as a badge of honor because it showed that you were tough, not weak like others. My childhood was complicated, messy, and dysfunctional. My family lived in a multi-generational home with my parents, siblings, grandparents, aunts, uncles, and cousins, so privacy was non-existent. There were frequent arguments, financial struggles, religious obligations, and each day was steeped in cultural, gender, and religious bias. Women were taught that our roles were to be those of a wife and a mother. Secondary education and working outside of the home were actively discouraged and seen as unproductive to the overall family dynamic. I recall that an aunt dared to work as a secretary in an office setting. My grandfather, the patriarch of the family, called her "rebellious" and "disobedient," and she was exiled from the rest of the family.*

*I quickly learned that it was easier to keep your head down and your mouth closed to keep the peace and survive. There was also frequent abuse in my home; physical abuse by my grandfather towards my grandmother, uncles, cousins, and even my siblings; verbal abuse showered in every direction but aimed mostly at the women and children; and sexual abuse at the hands of an older, male cousin towards myself and other female children in our home. The abuse became a routine, daily occurrence, despite my pleadings for it to stop. I was told that if I revealed it to any adults, I would be the one punished—or worse, that I would experience even more extreme trauma. About a year into this scenario, in an attempt to keep my younger female cousins and sister from experiencing this abuse, I struck a deal with my abuser and offered to take it all on myself. After all, pain and suffering were the norms in our home, so why should I complain now? This continued for several years until one day when my mother took me out for ice cream and asked me about the abuse that she was suspi-*

*cious of. I admitted that it was taking place, holding back on details and frequency. I saw the anger and pain in her eyes, so again tried to take on the responsibility and held back communicating my deepest thoughts and feelings about the experience. Instead, I felt the need to express to my mother that I was okay even though I wasn't. "I am okay, it wasn't that bad. Please, don't worry about me, mom, I will be fine." But I was not okay, I had died a little on the inside over those years, but I felt that I couldn't tell anyone how I felt and the pain I had experienced. At least now I could breathe a little. He had left, and I was still alive. Life goes on.*

*Years passed, and I stuffed down the emotional pain, excelled in high school, and moved on to college. I always knew that I wanted to graduate from college and have a meaningful career despite what I had been taught as a child. I wanted to prove my grandfather wrong and show the world that women are capable of anything and offer immense value to any industry. I had my share of boyfriends but never fully trusted any of them, always leading to short relationships. I was a terrible judge of character and thought I knew what I wanted in a relationship, things like physical and emotional safety. Still, my past experiences marred my perceptions of what a healthy relationship should look like. I had not seen healthy relationships modeled for me as a child, so determining what that should look like in my own life was impossible. I dated my fair share of men who took advantage of me personally, professionally, emotionally, and who cheated on me. Still, I lacked the self-confidence to stand up to them; instead I ended up as a tearful mess, which I took to be a reflection of something I had done wrong. Thankfully, all that changed when I met my husband. Suddenly I met a man I instantly knew would be different. I quickly found out he was kind, funny, smart, trustworthy, empathetic, and best of all, he loved me for me, unconcerned about my past. He was unlike anyone else I had ever known, and through his love, I began to heal. I trusted him with my heart and soul and still do, 22 years later.*

*We married, had two children who became my entire world, and with great passion, I started a career managing health and social justice nonprofits. I took to this work like I was made for it and found myself moving up in the community, being sought after as an expert in fundraising and management, lobbying state leaders, attending board meetings, and excelling in my field. The irony of this is that while I could help vulnerable, oppressed, and ill people, I could not undo the trauma I experienced in my own life. I also managed, through over a dozen surgeries, the care of my son with congenital health issues. His medical care extended into three different states and almost required a degree in insurance advocacy and medical transcription to get him the attention needed for his conditions. Every day began at dawn and ended well past midnight, as I worked full time, cared for two small boys, and attended the daily therapies, treatments, and medical appointments with my youngest son. I also dealt with the cancer diagnosis of my mother-in-law, a family member's attempted suicides, and the death of friends and family. Through it all, I was a rock. People looked to me to be the strong one, offer advice, encouragement, hope. That was my role. I had to be okay.*

*Thirteen years ago, everything changed. While raising my family and working a full-time, stressful job, I developed food poisoning from a chicken salad sandwich: the fever, abdominal pain, vomiting, and diarrhea were so severe, I almost blacked out. Hours later, diarrhea turned to blood, and I couldn't leave the toilet. I honestly thought that I was dying, was barely able to talk, and lay shaking on the cold tiled bathroom floor. My husband rushed me to the regional hospital near our house. In the emergency room, a CT scan showed that my colon was so swollen and inflamed that they immediately transferred me via ambulance to a larger hospital downtown. I spent 3 days in the Intermediate Care Unit, receiving antibiotics, IV fluids, and pain meds. The diagnosis was unclear: the hospitalist said E. coli gastroenteritis, but the gastroenterologist said possible ulcerative colitis. A colonoscopy was recommended, but it couldn't be completed until I was better.*

*One month later, the pain and bloating with diarrhea continued, so I followed up with the GI specialist, hoping he could help. Sadly, that was not my experience:*

*Dr.: Hi, I'm Dr. Blah Blah. (Limp fish handshake) So, why are you here? (Looking at my chart and avoiding eye contact)*

*Me: (Sitting in a gown, shivering from waiting 30 minutes in the exam room) Hi, Doctor. Well, I recently was in the hospital for a bad case of E. coli. They recommended I follow up with you to have a colonoscopy for diagnosis and treatment. I still have pain and a lot of loose stool; I didn't know if that is normal or not.*

*Dr.: (Looking at the computer) Uh-huh, okay. (Silence) Well, you're too young for colon cancer, so it's probably nothing serious. I'll do one if you want. (Turns to me) Try some probiotics for the pain, and Kaopectate for loose stools. I will have the nurse set up the colonoscopy if you want one.*

*I couldn't believe it. "Really?" I thought. "You'll do a colonoscopy if I want one? Who WANTS a colonoscopy?! Shouldn't you make that call? Did you read my hospital record to see about possible colitis?" But I just sat there, startled, and wondered why I was in a gown if he didn't even do a physical exam.*

*Me: Uh, okay, so, that's it?*

*Dr.: (Already closing the door on his way out)*

*I had the colonoscopy, which is an experience that I will never forget. The colon prep process was a challenge from the chronic pain, bloating, and diarrhea, which was exacerbated by the Golytely, but I stuck to it, hopeful that it would lead to answers. I was prepped, and as I was rolled into the procedure room on the gurney, the last words I heard before the anesthetic took hold were from the gastroenterologist, who told the staff present, "Oh, good, this is the girl I was telling you about. The one who was bleeding from her ass." I turned my head to see his smug smile as I floated off to sleep. A few weeks passed, and I was dreading the follow-up appointment since our last encounter had gone so poorly. Nevertheless, I wanted to get to the bottom of this once and for all.*

*Dr.: (Talking as he entered the room, head down, reading my chart, and sitting on his rolling doctor stool.) So, everything looked fine. I took out two small polyps. There*

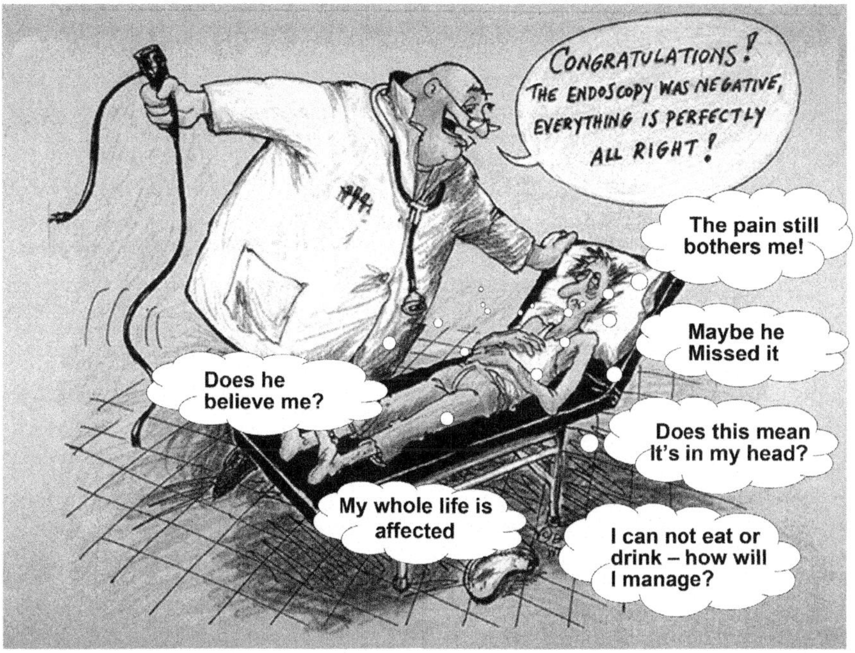


**Figure 22.** The colonoscopy was negative, so there is nothing wrong

*was very mild inflammation but nothing like ulcerative colitis or Crohn's disease and certainly no cancer. (Looks up) So, good news all around.*

*Me: Well, that's good. So why am I still having so much pain and loose bowel movements? Will that resolve on its own? Is it left over from the infection?*

*Dr.: (Looking at the computer and typing) Probably. Don't worry about it. Stress causes this, too, especially in women. You'll be fine. I won't need to see you again unless something changes. Just follow up with your primary care doc if needed. (Gets up and heads to the door) Take care.*

*It seemed to me he had no idea what was happening or what to do for me.*

*The entire encounter lasted less than 5 minutes. I couldn't believe that he dismissed my questions so quickly. His words stung like a slap on the face. He didn't need to see me, when I still felt so bad with these symptoms!? He had no interest in or understanding of what was happening and what it meant to me. He was really saying, "Your colonoscopy showed nothing relevant, so it's not that serious to me, and I don't want to spend any more time dealing with you." I was angry and frustrated.*

*As a young girl, I was taught not to question authority, and today, even as a grown, educated woman, I still tend to resort to this thinking and keep from voicing my true feelings. If a specialist did not think my symptoms were an issue, then maybe they weren't. Perhaps I was a baby. I felt embarrassed. My family's words echoed: "Suck it up, you're fine, stop making a big deal about it."* So, I thought, *"Okay, I'll just deal with it."*

*Over the next several years, I continued with abdominal pain and diarrhea. Still, it intensified and became almost constant, depending on the time of day and what I had eaten. I thought it was worse when I ate dairy or meat, so I eliminated them and other foods from my diet: broccoli, asparagus, dairy, beef, and pork. I tried heating pads, sleeping with a pillow under my rib cage, Gas-X pills, Imodium, and upwards of 12 probiotic pills a day.*

*The effects on my family over the years were profound. I had to cancel on friends and family events frequently because of the symptoms. I wasn't well and didn't know if I could get to a bathroom quickly enough or eat the food offered. I missed family soccer games, college football games, concerts, and barbeques. I spent the weekends mostly in bed, and my husband and kids played games or watched movies downstairs. My marriage was affected; who wants to be intimate when dealing with constant pain, restricted diets, and unpredictable bowel habits? Things were getting worse, despite my best efforts to self-manage. I didn't know what to do, so I relented and saw three other doctors, who, after reviewing my chart, told me that I should eat more yogurt (but I gave up dairy because it made my pain worse), drink more water (novel idea, why didn't I think of that?!), try yoga (is there a bathroom nearby?). Maybe I should hike or swim to reduce stress (if it were just that easy, with what free time?).*

*I had given up hope that a gastroenterologist was going to help me, so in the last effort to find answers, I saw an internist. This was my worst interaction:*

*Dr.: Could you be exaggerating the severity of the pain a bit? From what I see in your chart, there is no structural cause for your symptoms. If it were as bad as you say, how can you hold a job or raise a family? Women can get hysterical and exaggerate pain, especially at certain times of the month. Maybe it's not as bad as you say?*

*Stunned, pinching my arm to keep from crying and embarrassing myself, I felt the need to justify myself and my symptoms. My inner voice screamed: "Why are you letting someone speak to you like this, make you feel insignificant and unworthy, and even call you a liar?" Yet the little girl in me needed to prove to him that I was strong enough to manage my symptoms while proving the legitimacy of my pain and its effect on my life. I told him that I worked every day, even though I was hurting, with a heating pad hiding under my desk. I cared for my family, even when repeatedly going to the bathroom, to try to give them a happy childhood, and that I served on eight different nonprofit committees and boards in town, serving my community all while discreetly eating Imodium like candy. He didn't seem to care.*

*I decided that to better my career choices and provide legitimacy for my work with my son, I needed to get a master's degree. I began my MEd program while working full time and trying desperately to keep my symptoms from worsening. Despite my best efforts, my pain was now widespread and had also begun to affect my joints, hands, and feet. I was always tired, living on caffeine, and developed brain fogginess and forgetfulness. The rheumatologist said I had fibromyalgia and gave me gabapentin for*

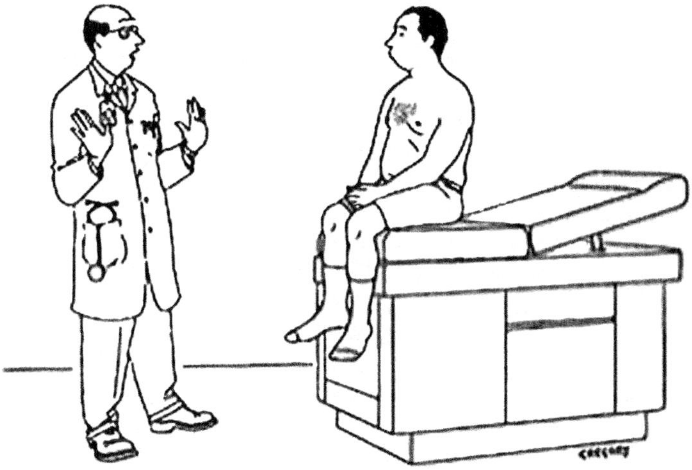

**"Whoa – <u>way</u> too much information !"**

**Figure 23.** When doctors lose interest

*the pain and sleep. I was frustrated. Is fibromyalgia a real diagnosis, and is it related to the GI symptoms? Did it all come from the damn chicken salad sandwich? Did I do something to cause this? I felt at the end of my rope, hopeless, and lost. I had lost over 15 pounds and was taking 1,800 mg of gabapentin and a handful of probiotics and Imodium each day just to be able to function.*

*Over time, I began to miss work when my symptoms were severe and flaring. I even had to leave an awards dinner early, where I was honored as a top Professional Under 40. On the ride home, I sat in the car with tears in my eyes, frustrated and tired at the course my health had taken all these years.*

*I wanted to scream: "I AM IN PAIN. WHAT IS WRONG WITH ME? WHY CAN'T SOMEONE HELP ME!" I felt the diagnosis of fibromyalgia, the probiotics, yogurt, water, yoga were all hodge-podge recommendations given as a last resort. I couldn't bear to hear that I had "mystery" symptoms or that I was "exaggerating." I believed that my doctors were saying, "We don't know what else to tell you, and we don't see any legitimate reason for your symptoms, so this is the best we can do. We don't want to really understand how this is affecting your life. So, please, stop coming; Figure it out on your own." My medical chart must have said: "She is exaggerating the pain and diarrhea, and probably won't accept that this is stress. Smile, nod, and send her on her way with a new probiotic to try."*

*So, I stopped seeing doctors and tried to cope and adapt my life to this "new normal." I got my MEd with honors, poured my energy into my work and my family, and did the best I could to manage my symptoms. This was just the way life was going to be. Then, suddenly, after 17 years with the same company, my husband was offered a job transfer across the country. We accepted, looking for new opportunities and a change of pace. This is when my life changed. I too, started a new job with a nonprofit called the Rome Foundation that I was excited about, mostly because it focused on GI disorders. "Well, I know a little something about that," I thought! I was suddenly working with the best gastroenterologists in the world, but I certainly wasn't going to ask them about my symptoms. That was unprofessional, and the likelihood that they could even help seemed remote, at best. However, while out for dinner, after stumbling back to the table from the bathroom for the third time, my husband convinced me to make an appointment with Dr. Drossman, one of the physicians I worked with.*

*Dr. Drossman: (Looking directly at me with a smile) Hello. Thanks for coming in. How are you, and how can I help?*

*Okay, right away, I thought, "Why is he looking at me instead of the computer?!"*

*Me: Uh, well, I have some stomach issues and thought maybe you could help.*

*Dr.: Okay, glad to try to help. (smile) Tell me about your symptoms.*

*This dialogue went on for about an hour. With his encouragement, I discussed my symptoms, my feelings about them, and their effect on my family. He asked follow-up questions, expressed empathy: concern and support for my feelings and the impact my symptoms had on my personal life. I was a little bit excited. I thought to myself, "Why had I never experienced this dialogue with a doctor before?"*

*Suddenly a glimmer of hope began in my soul. Even if he couldn't completely help me, I knew he cared and was willing to try. I felt validated and supported but was overwhelmed. When he told me that post-infection IBS caused my symptoms and could be treated, I was relieved. Through his explanations and diagrams, I learned*

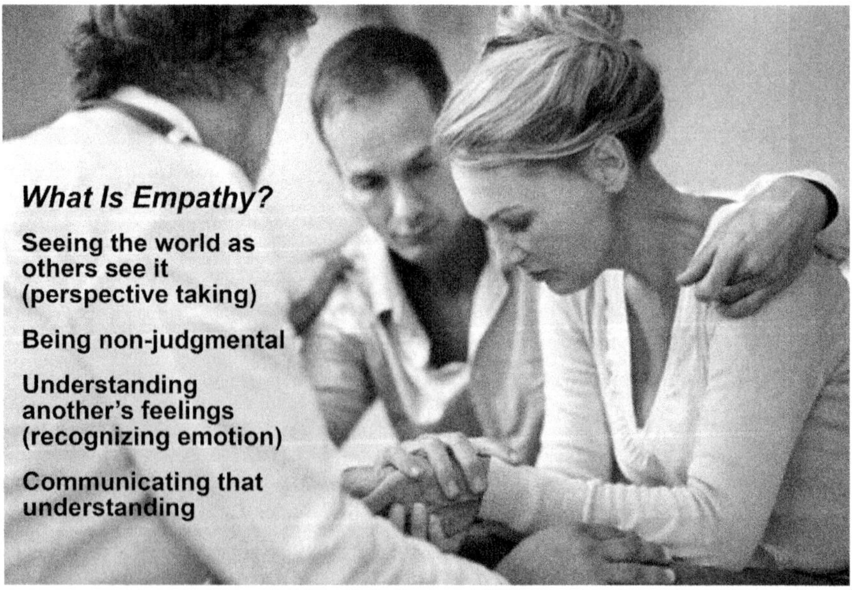


Figure 24. Empathy

*that post-infection IBS could occur when there is a gastrointestinal infection associated with stress. Strangely, this was exciting to hear, as it was so validating. I had never received a diagnosis before! I also learned how my earlier experiences triggered my helplessness in managing this illness, and more than likely made me more prone to them in the first place. Then we talked through treatment options. Dr. Drossman explained why he would like to use an antibiotic for the IBS and an antidepressant to treat the brain's poor regulation of the pain. Then he asked how I felt about the plan, and we discussed the risks and benefits. I agreed willingly, as I was now part of the process of my care. While recovery could take time, he assured me that he was in it for the long term, and I knew he wouldn't abandon me.*

*They say that when one is heard, they feel valued and loved. This was certainly the case for me, especially after so many years of being ignored and dismissed.*

*Today, my GI pain is resolved. I normally eat without restriction but still don't have a taste for pork or much dairy. I do have occasional flare-ups of nausea, bloating, and even diarrhea sometimes, but they are quickly resolved with over-the-counter treatments now. I also use psychological interventions to manage my symptoms, such as diaphragmatic breathing techniques, visualization, and techniques like reframing and understanding that things won't necessarily spin out of control; and if they do, I have the skill set to handle what comes my way. I am now able to pinpoint the cause of my flares—mostly stressors such as work, family, or the occasional pandemic—and work to calm my brain to calm my gut's response. Thanks to the neuromodulator I took, my widespread pain is gone. My ability to regulate pain anywhere in my body is functioning normally now. How did this happen? Was it the pills or a placebo effect? Was it the doctor or just the passage of time? Or was it me?*

*Here's what I now know:*

*The patient-doctor relationship is complex and challenging. Chronic illness and pain can make you feel like you are spiraling out of control, especially when you falsely assume there isn't any "real" cause for it and seemingly no way to treat it. Patients see a doctor hoping to regain control through treatment but know they may not have a "quick fix." What patients want is honest dialogue, to be heard and understood, and not dismissed. They don't mind if a doctor says they aren't sure what's going on, as long as they are committed to finding out, and won't abandon them.*

*My care changed when I was able to honestly share my symptoms, thoughts, and feelings with Dr. Drossman and know that he would listen and try to help; that made me feel validated and empowered. Even on days when I don't feel 100%, I know that, together, we will come up with a plan to address my symptoms. Knowing that he wants my input lets me know I can trust him, and that makes me compliant with the treatments that we decide on together.*

*My interaction with my doctor helped me to find my voice and to advocate for myself. Through this ordeal, I understood what my participation had been in the negative interactions with doctors. The difficulties I had with them reverberated and amplified the feelings of helplessness, lack of control, and anger that came from my childhood traumas. So, while I ferociously fought for my children, family, and friends, I retreated when the doctors came at me. I am still a work in progress. It is unrealistic to think that a patient with chronic illness and a history of trauma and abuse can overcome past coping mechanisms and unhealthy psychological mindsets overnight.*

*I also have a better understanding of what is happening inside my body. Education is a powerful tool for patients and can help them understand the role that diet, stress, trauma, and other external factors play in their illness and their recovery. I also have a better understanding of the role the brain plays in chronic illnesses. There is a powerful connection between the body and the brain, and treatments should complement them both to achieve total symptom management. Health psychologists are an excellent addition to the treatment plan for any patient experiencing GI disorders, and learning how to identify and manage the triggers that exacerbate your symptoms is an important part of the self-management process.*

*No one should be given the power to take my health, my light, or my truth. I now feel a new sense of empowerment, as a patient and as a professional woman. For the first time, I can say, yes, I am okay. Really, truly, okay.*

### *Issues That Affected My Treatment*

My illness and recovery generated many thoughts and feelings. They influenced me to find out why so many patients similarly afflicted also feel helpless in their role as a patient and in their interactions with their doctors, as I experienced. This experience has led me to find the answers and to use this knowledge to help others as a patient advocate.

I found that many issues affect treatment for patients; there are quite a few things to consider. Unfortunately, medical care in the US is draped in societal, gender, racial, and religious biases that have a powerful impact on the care we receive. These issues drive so many patients with DGBI to have such a negative patient experience, and ultimately, poor outcomes—just as they drove my treatment (and my life, really) until I met Dr. Drossman, who validated my illness experience and empowered me to take control of my health journey.

**Gender stereotyping.** Even in 2020, gender stereotyping is still a driving issue in healthcare outcomes. Women have been socially conditioned for generations to "be nice," "ask nicely," and "wait our turn" when it comes to seeking medical care; ultimately, this works against us. I used to hear myself say things like, "I am sorry to bother you, I know you are busy and probably have patients who are sicker than I am, but could you please help me?" About a decade ago, I was traveling with a male colleague and two female colleagues to visit volunteers in a neighboring city several hours away. After just a few miles out onto the highway, our rental car suddenly jerked and sputtered to a stop and suddenly began spewing hot oil and air conditioning coolant through the vents, covering our faces, bodies, and clothes, and burning our eyes and skin immediately. We sat stunned for a minute, and when we realized that we were developing chemical burns, we called 911 to get to the nearby hospital. When we arrived, it was evident that we needed medical care. Since my male colleague had been the driver and I had been the front-seat passenger, we had inhaled the coolant and were developing burns inside our nose and mouth. We both had the same injuries and reported the same symptoms, levels of pain, and severity of symptoms, but my male colleague was taken into triage and seen immediately. At the same time, I was escorted to a gurney in the hallway of the ER for 3 hours without being offered a gown and was given only a few paper towels to wipe off excess chemicals from my stained clothing and body. I asked nurses passing by multiple times for help, only to be told that all personnel were busy, and that I would need to keep waiting. My eyes, nose, and throat burned like fire; and my breathing was labored with frequent coughing and wheezing. My chest, arms, and face were red and covered with tiny blisters, but I continued to wait. From my gurney, I could see down the hallway and into the room where my male colleague was receiving care, had been cleaned up, and was resting. I couldn't believe it. The attending physician came to see me just when I had finally tried to clean myself up in the restroom, and, not finding me, he went on, leaving me waiting for another 4 hours. I was finally treated and released, needing follow-up care for several months because my injuries were not treated as quickly as my colleague's had been.

**Pain management.** Gender stereotyping also leads to the belief that emotional rather than physical causes lead to women's pain, even when clinical tests show their physical nature.[41, 42] Recently, I consulted with a female urogynecology surgeon after having several years of worsening gynecological pain and dysfunction. She recommended that I have pelvic floor surgery. One week after having the rectocele and cystocele repair, I developed severe pain. I went back to the gynecologist's office for a checkup and removal of the catheter I had come home with. I was not my best self, wearing Tinkerbell PJ pants, a hoodie, and having just rolled out of bed, in a massive amount of pain. Despite my insistence that something was not right, she did not examine me. My husband who was with me saw that the staff was not taking my request seriously. He intervened, insisting that they examine me or at least give me better pain medication. Despite both our efforts, I was instead told somewhat sarcastically, by an attending female physician, that even "... 78-year-old women have the same procedure without much postoperative pain." I was told that nothing was wrong, was offered ibuprofen and gabapentin, and was sent home. A few days later, I awoke in severe pain and contemplated calling an ambulance. Instead, I called to see another physician who, based on the same report of severe pain, examined me and discovered that I had an internal ulcer from a ruptured stitch that had become infected. Then I was treated appropriately, and the pain was quickly resolved. This illustrates how the belief that women exaggerate their pain affects proper pain management, even from female physicians toward female patients. Sadly, it is no surprise. Studies show that females' pain is often minimized and mocked and that they are coaxed into silence.[41, 43] Doctors tend to underdiagnose and undertreat women, leading to adverse healthcare outcomes.[44, 45] Comedian Wanda Sykes, in a recent comedy special, shared her own experience with this kind of treatment after her mastectomy for a breast cancer diagnosis. She was not offered any postoperative pain medications, told that ibuprofen would be enough to manage her pain from surgery because women—particularly women of color—are more prone to exaggerate their reports of pain and to opioid addiction. She commented that while she was recovering from a major operation, taking Advil, her male friends were given Percocet to treat an infected hangnail. That doesn't quite seem equitable. Similarly, and without proper evidence, doctors may incorrectly diagnose women with chronic pain as having a mental health condition and are more likely to prescribe psychotropic drugs.[43, 46] If you are a woman, chances are that you have experienced some degree of this—which leads us to the next impact: how this affects us, the patients.

**Impact on the patient.** When you ask a woman with chronic pain about her illness experience, you will often hear stories of guilt, shame, embarrassment, and even depression. From my experience I have learned that women are naturally vulnerable to becoming unnecessarily self-critical and often feel frustrated, angry, and socially isolated when dealing with pain or chronic illness.[43, 45] Chronic illness can also impair our ability to work, care for loved ones, interact with others, and perform basic personal tasks. With IBS, concerns about bowel habits impact dating, intimacy, and sexuality, creating further isolation.[30, 45, 46] This leads us to feel stigmatized by family, friends, co-workers, and retreat even more. We shouldn't expect to feel stigmatized by our doctors, too. Sadly, many of us do.

**Stigma from doctors.** When doctors stigmatize patients who have symptoms such as those of DGBI, the impact on the patient is profound. If you accept the diagnosis from a dualistic perspective, you may develop feelings of guilt and self-blame for having a condition not perceived as "real." Telling patients—or inferring—that they are "crazy," "hysterical," or "unstable" disengages them. When doctors said I was exaggerating the severity of my symptoms, I felt delegitimized and stigmatized, stemming from the implication that I was "crazy." About 50% of IBS patients do not tell their family members and friends about being diagnosed with these disorders because they are afraid of being misunderstood or not believed.[45] This sense of isolation and stigma increases the stress we feel as we attempt to manage these illnesses on our own. For further information on understanding this concept and its impact on patients, please go to **https://romedross.video/StigmaIBS**.

**The role of stress.** The role of stress on symptom severity in chronic illness is well studied and documented. However, when physicians tell patients that their illness is the result of stress, it implies a single cause, which we now know is not scientifically based. Importantly, it also leads to the patient feeling in some way responsible. They feel helpless as to how to stop it, angry at the insinuation that they are to blame for the illness because they lack good stress management and have no realistic options to change their stress response. When a doctor told me to manage my stress better, I remember thinking, "Sure, got it. So, I will quit my job, divorce my husband, put my kids up for adoption, and move to a deserted island!" Doctors often struggle to reframe this perspective. Properly validating and accepting the idea that stress plays a role for the patient requires doctors to explain the bidirectionality of stress and GI symptoms. The brain-gut axis illuminates how chronic and severe symptoms can cause psychological distress, which in turn affects the severity and chronicity of the illness. DGBI are *not* a psychiatric illness.[31] Explanations like this can be very enlightening for patients. The explanation certainly opened my mind to listen to my doctor's suggestion for stress management, including the use of a neuromodulator.[30, 31]

**The power of a physical examination.** A physical examination can make you feel validated because it is a demonstration that the doctor is committed to engaging with you in the effort to diagnose. In the last 10 years, I can count on one hand the number of times that a doctor performed a physical examination. It profoundly impacted my perception of the doctor's concern for me, and their interest and understanding of my symptoms. It enabled a much-needed connection.[47] Communicating confidence, a sense of security, and trust, change the dynamics of the visit. You are likely to feel more connected to the doctor, to trust their diagnosis and proposed treatment, and to want to continue to engage with them.[48] We as patients are open to education about our condition once this connection is established.

**Patient education.** The Latin word for *doctor* is *docere,* which means *to teach.* Since I'm a former teacher, I love that this word conveys that doctors are in the perfect role to not only diagnose and treat but to also educate patients about their conditions and treatment options. Patients want to be educated, and if doctors don't give us the information we need, we'll seek it from less reliable sources (like Dr. Google).

Twenty years ago, patient education meant handing out "dumbed down" pamphlets in the office. Now, we patients do not want to be talked down to. We want scientifically backed education that is relevant and complete.[45, 48] The best and most effective form of education is in the office, one-on-one, with a doctor or clinical care team member, having a dialogue and then using diagrams to show mechanisms of action, physiology, and the rationale for treatment. No matter what type of education a doctor chooses, frequent checks are needed to ensure correct understanding along the way.[30, 41] This interactive learning environment creates the opportunity for improved understanding, shared decision making, and treatment adherence. It also motivates the patient to take back some control and develop self-management strategies.[30, 49, 50]

**Set the follow-up appointment.** Patients in pain do not want to be abandoned. Particularly when the condition is chronic, the doctor should set up a return appointment for you. Until I met Dr. Drossman, I was only told that I should return if needed; there was no long-term plan of care. When the doctor initiates a plan for ongoing care, they communicate a commitment to your well-being, which sets the stage for positive interactions going forward.[48]

**Ditching the shame.** Much of my childhood experience left me feeling tremendous shame, which happened again when I became chronically ill. I have learned a great deal from Dr. Brené Brown on how to overcome and heal that feeling, which derived from my past traumas. She says this about shame: "*Shame blocks vulnerability. Identifying and naming shame is essential so that we do not get stuck in thinking, 'I'm not worthy of love and belonging' but can shift out of shame into a deep knowing that we are all worthy of love and belonging no matter what. Understanding shame means identifying and naming shame as soon as we feel it, so that we don't get stuck in a 'shame storm.' Since shame cannot stand being spoken, it can be liberating to understand shame and find a friend to talk to when feeling stuck in shame. The antidote to shame is empathy. Empathy is all about feeling understood and knowing that we are not alone.*"

Doesn't this just give you goosebumps?! I love how this illustrates how patients can overcome the shame and stigma that we might feel about our illness only by talking about it and finding a sense of empathy with others. We all need to know that we belong and that we are understood and accepted, even with our complicated pasts, traumas, flaws, and illnesses. It's not easy to be vulnerable, to reach out to a stranger and ask for help or advice. It's not easy to tell your story. Let's face it, who wants to talk about personal issues, or worse, talk about poop?! I assure you, though, that the benefits of vulnerability and sharing far outweigh the negatives. I have learned that by telling my personal story, I can provide help and hope to others facing similar issues, all while speaking life to myself, healing past pains, and better managing my own health. This is a part of our self-management, our self-actualization, and our self-care. Change will not happen overnight, so be gentle with yourself and continue to take the steps outlined here to help you take back your control, your voice, and your health journey.

**Hopeful, not hopeless.** Finally, we all need hope. I hear from so many patients about their sense of hopelessness in the face of their illness experiences. It seems to them that no one understands their illness, treatments are fleeting and somewhat unreliable, and so their recovery is unachievable. I believe that hope involves resetting achievable expectations. Chronic illness is just that: chronic. There is no magic wand to wave and bring about complete and total recovery. However, as you can begin to understand more about your diagnosis, implement the available treatments, and understand the role that you have in advocating for and managing your journey, you can achieve small steps forward to a life of more normalcy and joy. Hopefulness also involves sharing your concerns and fears with others so you know you are not alone, and solutions can be achieved together. I love hearing from patients facing the same struggles that I have faced because I am able to offer them hope, friendship, and someone who understands and will listen. Often, that is therapeutic enough. We are all in this together!

If you need someone to reach out to who truly understands, you are always welcome to connect with me. Find me on Twitter @JohannahRuddy.

### *The Doctor's Perspective on Johannah's Experience*[31] *—Douglas A. Drossman, MD*

Johannah's remarkable story reflects a transition from illness to health, and from helplessness to self-efficacy. It started with a bacterial (*E. coli*) gastroenteritis occurring during a time of intense stress. This co-occurrence was the basis for developing post-infection IBS.[51, 52] She was treated appropriately for the severe pain and bloody diarrhea during the acute infection; why, then, did her medical experience deteriorate after the infection resolved? As we've discussed, when abnormal tests were present, the symptoms were considered more legitimate. But when the colonoscopy and other tests became negative, there was no "disease" to explain the symptoms, and that imposed psychological stigma.[8] Furthermore, these days the healthcare system reimburses doctors to do more tests and focus their time on "sicker" patients. This may have led doctors to allocate less time and attention to Johannah, despite her disabling symptoms and reduced quality of life.[1] Finally, doctors not familiar with the diagnosis and treatment of DGBI may feel unknowledgeable, ineffective, or inadequate to treat them. They may even believe that patients with these disorders don't fall within their medical responsibility. Then, when confronted with having to care for them, they may behave in ways that are perceived by patients as dismissive or even stigmatizing.

There are two sides to understanding how this story evolved. What about Johannah's contribution to this process? She grew up in the '70s and '80s, when family culture and societal factors[53, 54] encouraged stoicism and gender role socialization.[55] As she describes, girls were taught not to be assertive and were to submit to authority (male, in particular) without question. The trauma she experienced further limited her sense of control to handle unwanted situations like illness, increased her vulnerability, and also reduced trust in those with authority.[32] Furthermore, the stress of this all only worsened her pain and her ability to adapt.[32, 56]

My research has demonstrated that early trauma does not cause DGBI. However, it impacts individuals who later deal with GI illness: on the severity of the symptoms, on personal attitudes and perceptions of their capability to deal with them, and the resultant patient behaviors toward healthcare providers. I also found from the research that feelings of helplessness, shame, lack of trust, and stigmatization generated at the time of the trauma, "reverberate" when the patient is later confronted by new challenging situations, like GI illness.[32] So the attributions patients make about their current illness derive from what they incorporated during the earlier trauma experience.

This helps to explain why Johannah could not effectively advocate for herself when she was treated poorly by her physicians but was very capable of promoting her family's interests. The effects she described of her early adverse experiences led to an inability to interact with her physicians effectively, creating the perfect storm: a vicious cycle of dissatisfaction, helplessness, and suffering. As a result, she gave up on the medical system.

How did this cycle reverse? During her first visit, I gave her a diagnosis and explained why she had her symptoms. I responded to her concerns, which legitimized them, explained the possible treatments that could follow, and emphasized that she would make the care decisions. I offered to work collaboratively and to be available whatever the outcome of any treatment plan. I served as her advisor and promoted a patient-centered care model that lifted her emotional distress, increased her trust and self-efficacy, and empowered her to regain control. In her words: *"My care changed when I was able to honestly share my symptoms, thoughts, and feelings with my doctor and know that he was going to listen and try to help; that made me feel validated and empowered."* The vicious cycle reversed, and Johannah no longer feels helpless when seeing doctors. She is now capable of encouraging them to engage in the way she expects, which benefits them both. To hear and see Johannah's story, go to **http://bit.ly/2wAT96l**.

Furthermore, this personal growth began a new career for her as a patient advocate and educator in the field. From her experiences and her innate sense of what patients encounter, she can help them to find solutions. She has parlayed her skills into social media channels and educational programs for patients. She is successful in obtaining educational grants and has evolved an academic career writing peer-reviewed publications. I'm pleased to say that we now partner on developing and implementing learning programs to teach these values to doctors and patients. This book is a result of this collaboration.

## The Patient-Doctor Relationship—A Two-Way Street

Communication is a two-way street, so the PDR is a two-way street. Patients and doctors each have a role, and they both need to fulfill these different roles to develop patient-centered care.

Table 2 shows what patients and doctors should know.

*Table 2. What Patients and Doctors Should Know*[30]

| Patients should know | Doctors should know |
|---|---|
| You and your health are worth fighting for, no matter what. | Patients need to feel that you care about them as a person and not feel judged. |
| You can demand to be treated with dignity and respect. | Patients need to feel respected to share personal details that will assist you in their care. |
| You have a right to share your personal thoughts and feelings about your care. | Patients need to feel that their doctor will be receptive to their thoughts and feelings. |
| You have a right to ask questions and receive visual aids to understand your diagnosis and treatment. | Patients need to understand the diagnosis and treatment plan so they can participate and feel like they have a say in the process. |
| You have a right to be heard. | Patients are not impressed with ego and prestige; they want you to be humane and to care about the impact of the illness on their life. |
| You have the right to engage with your doctor as a partner. | Patients are okay with "I don't know," so long as you continue to work with them or guide them to someone who will. |
| You can refuse treatment or seek another opinion if your needs are not being met. | Patients need to know that you are not going to abandon them. |

## Key Elements That Optimize the PDR

Now that we have described what a patient-centered PDR should look like, let's discuss the elements that make it work. As we keep emphasizing, both the doctor and the patient have a role in this. So, first, we will discuss the doctor's role—then look at what the patient needs to do.

### *The Doctor's Role*

Your doctor should be able to communicate with you in a way that enhances the PDR and facilitates patient-centered care.[39, 50] We offer ten tips for doctors to use, as seen in the video: **https://romedross.video/Q_A_10tips**:

- **listen actively**
- identify agenda(s)
- empathize
- validate feelings
- set realistic goals
- educate
- reassure
- negotiate
- "be there"

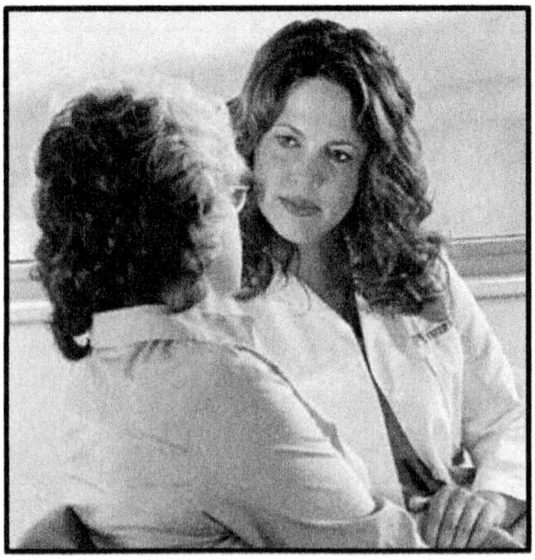

**Listen actively.** Many of us feel we are good listeners but are we? Consider being at a social reception with a friend or family member. You are standing together, maybe having a drink, and talking about your respective families. You both seem actively engaged as your partner discusses the children. You start thinking of your children. If at that moment I came over and asked you what your partner was saying, would you be surprised that you do not know? During conversations, sometimes we internally "take a break" from engaging in what is said to collect our thoughts before it is our turn to speak. Similarly, the doctor may be distracted during an office visit because they are sorting out a series of diagnostic questions to ask, typing the information into the electronic health record on the computer, and maybe even thinking about dinner plans that evening. You may notice that the doctor is not looking at you. Or perhaps they ask questions that seem unrelated to what you just said. With active listening, the doctor needs to engage fully, and with good eye contact. To fully understand your symptoms, thoughts, and feelings, doctors asking a question need to wait without interrupting. Then they construct the next set of questions based on what you say, rather than from a preset list.

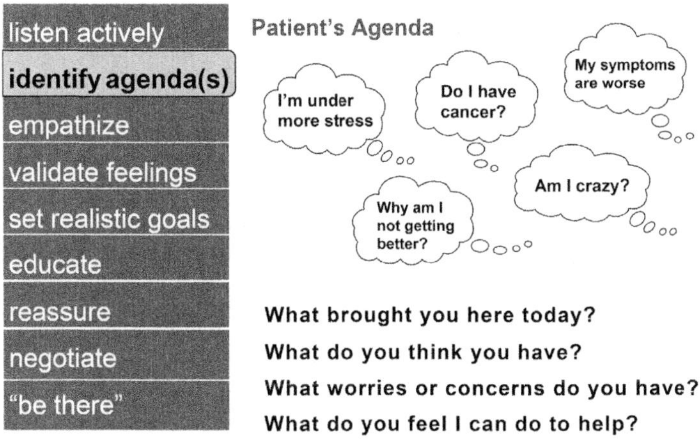


**Understand your agenda.** The doctor needs to find out the essential issues to discuss and can ask directly: "What would you like us to discuss today?" But setting the agenda also means knowing why you are coming, how *you* perceive your illness, what your concerns are, and how it all affects your life. The first visit is critical for setting the agenda for diagnosis and ongoing care. I've recommended that doctors ask four questions:

a. *What brought you here today?* You may have many reasons for requesting an office visit. They may be as straightforward as *"My stomach hurts,"* or more complicated, *"I need disability,"* or the reason may even be unconscious: *"This is the first anniversary of my father's death, and he had chest pain just like me."*
b. *What do you think you have?* Patients hold personal beliefs or concepts that often come from families and cultures. Understanding them can be used to help shape the treatment plan. It's not uncommon for patients with abdominal pain for many years to believe they have an undiagnosed infection despite negative diagnostic studies. Knowing the patient's beliefs can help shape the response. For example, I might say to a patient that the pain may have started with an infection that is no longer present, but it sensitized the nerves to continue to cause pain (similar to "phantom limb"). That would then allow for treatments directed toward a DGBI with visceral hypersensitivity.
c. *What worries or concerns do you have?* Patients often worry about cancer or other dangerous conditions but may be uncomfortable to volunteer this. Yet doctors may intuitively know from the clinical visit and the diagnostic studies that there is no cancer, and routinely reassure by saying, *"everything is okay."* However, this may not register with the patient because they did not articulate that concern. However, if the doctor asks the patient what concerns or worries they have, it offers the opportunity for the patient to express their concerns, which then leads to a realistic degree of reassurance. So, for example, I might say: *"Based on today's evaluation and the diagnostic studies, you do not have*

*evidence of cancer. The CT scan was negative 6 months ago, and you have had this pain for years. If the pain you have had for so many years was from cancer, we would have seen it on the x-ray. Nevertheless, I will stay vigilant and reconsider the diagnosis in the future if anything changes."* To view an example of a dialog addressing a patient with concerns about cancer, see: **http://bit.ly/2vmWWqF**.

d. *What do you feel I can do to help?* With this question, the doctor offers the patient the option to discuss expectations for their care. Some patients with chronic illness over many years may hold unrealistic beliefs: to be cured or pain-free. But the doctor can then reset expectations to a more realistic level (see below).

**Empathize.** Your doctor validates you when they say things like, *"I can see how difficult it has been to manage with your pain."* They should empathize with you, learn your perspective (how you see the world and your illness), be nonjudgmental, recognize and understand your feelings, and communicate their understanding of what you tell them. See Dr. Brené Brown's discussion of empathy in this video: **http://bit.ly/2Ms6Dwk**.

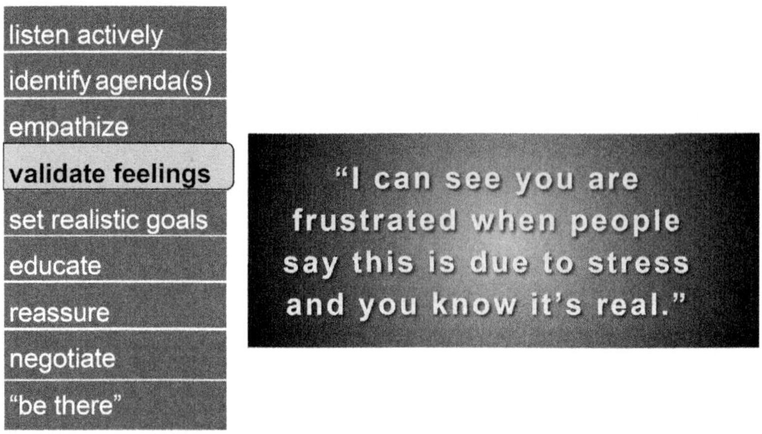


**Validate.** Even if the doctor does not agree with your perspective, it helps for them to provide an air of openness and acceptance.[57] Their recognition of your thoughts and feelings validates those thoughts and feelings. For example, if you are upset because others have said that your problem is just due to stress, the doctor can say, *"I can see you are upset when people say this is due to stress, and you know it's real."* Validating statements open the door to more dialogue about the role of stress in illness.

**Set realistic goals.** It is understandable for patients with chronic illness to want a rapid diagnosis and a cure. At the same time, the doctor may see the need to focus on ongoing management with realistic expectations for a good outcome. These differences need to be reconciled. For example, the doctor could say, *"I understand how much you want these symptoms to go away, but they are long-standing, and we therefore need to reset our expectations. If we can reduce your symptoms by 30% over the next several months, would that help?"*

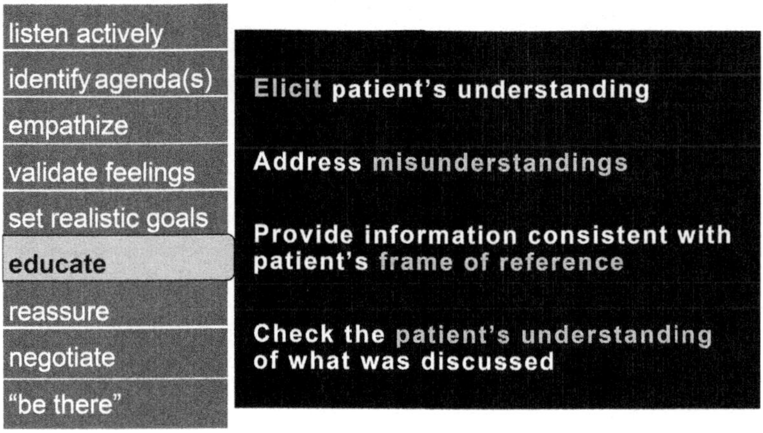


**Educate.** Education is therapeutic. The first visit is critical to providing proper knowledge about your condition and the plan of care. Numerous times I've heard patients say, "Nobody has told me that." I believe they have been told but in a manner that is brief or superficial so that it doesn't register. Providing education is an iterative process that includes checking on the patient's understanding, addressing any misconceptions, informing in a way that is consistent with the patient's knowledge of the illness, and making sure that their understanding matches up with what is said. These days illustrations, diagrams, and even videos are readily available. See the Rome Foundation's library of educational videos for patients: **https://theromefoundation.org/patient-educational-q-a/**. When you and the doctor are clear about your condition and the treatment you mutually decide upon, you will feel in more control of your symptoms and be able to participate in your long-term healthcare as a team member.

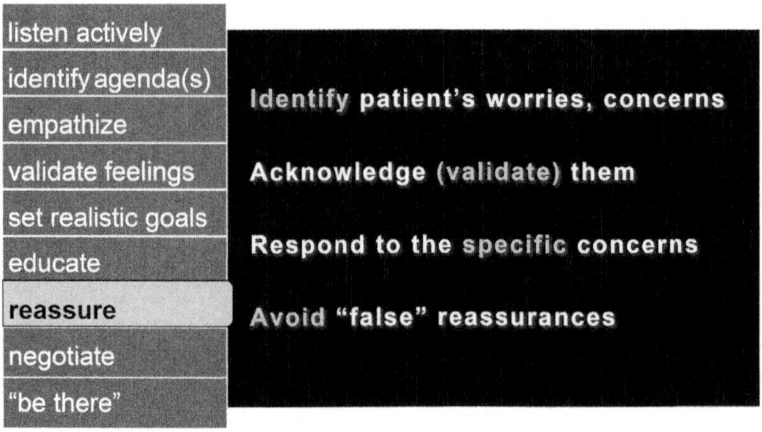


**Reassure.** Just like providing education, reassurance is an iterative process. It's not just a pat on the back, saying, *"Don't worry about it."* When done prematurely, reassurance is invalidating. Instead, the doctor must identify and acknowledge any concerns and then appropriately respond to them to validate them.

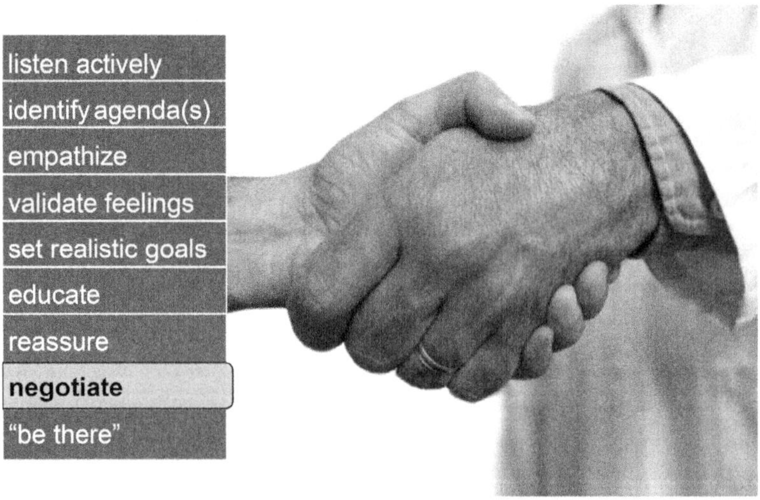


**Negotiate.** You and the doctor need to agree on diagnostic and treatment options. After educating you on treatment options, the doctor should elicit your personal experience, understanding, and interest in these options and provide you with choices (rather than directives) that are consistent with your expectations. For example, I usually give a patient several treatment options, stating the possible benefits and side effects. Then, we discuss the pros and cons of each treatment. We then work together to prioritize a sequential treatment plan. In this way, if on the next visit, if the response is less than ideal, we can go to the next step.

**Help the patient take responsibility.** Research has shown that patients with chronic illness do best when they take responsibility for their care, and doctors must encourage this. For example, instead of saying: *"How is your pain doing?"* I will say to my patient: *"How are you managing with your pain?"* The second question encourages the patient to take an active role in the management of their illness and reduces pressure on doctors to take more responsibility than needed. Doctors should offer you several treatment approaches, with a discussion of their risks and benefits, so that you can make an informed and thoughtful decision.

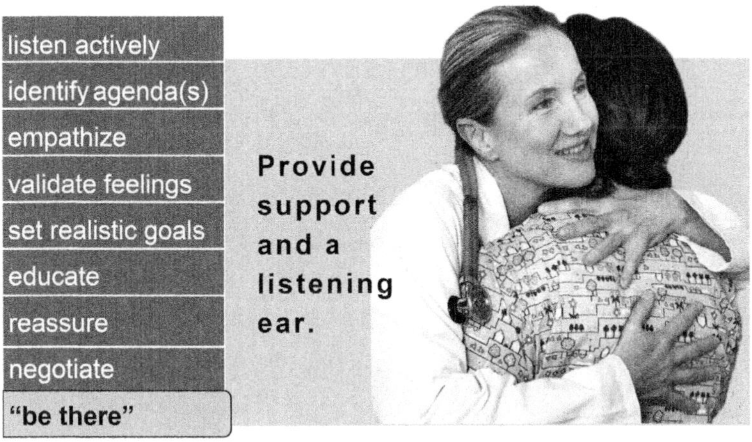


**Be there.** Providing support and a listening ear is indispensable for excellent communication and the PDR. It can be hard to reveal sensitive information, but it all pivots on the level of trust that emerges between doctor and patient. Though intense emotional issues may at first seem unrelated, they can impact the GI illness by lowering the pain threshold and adds to the emotional distress. Both factors increase the severity of the symptoms. So the doctor needs to have that information, as it may lead to more effective treatments. For example, my research has demonstrated a strong association between early trauma with the present severity of GI pain and other symptoms.[32] Negative emotions of helplessness, vulnerability, lack of trust, and anxiety that originated from the traumatic experiences "reverberate" later in life. They occur with new and challenging experiences where the patient again feels no sense of control. Chronic and severe GI illness is one example, and knowledge of relevant information about the past provides the opportunity for selecting brain-gut psychological treatments that will improve the GI symptoms and associated emotions. This video demonstrates how addressing early trauma can be sensitively elicited during the clinic visit: **https://romedross.video/ChangTopics**.

*Body Language—Nonverbal Communication—*
*It's not what you say but how you say it*

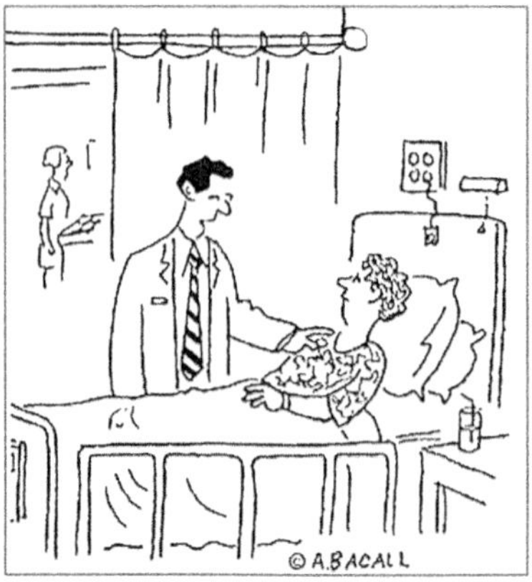


**"Of course I'm listening to your expression of spiritual suffering. Don't you see me making eye contact, striking an open posture, leaning towards you and nodding empathetically?"**

**Figure 25.** Nonverbal communication

Many years ago, I was supervising a nervous medical student interviewing a male teenager. The student didn't listen very much. Instead, he kept sneaking a glance at his small list of questions to try to get them all asked; his manner was quite stilted. The teenager looked down and seemed bored. A few minutes into the interview, the student's pager went off. He excused himself and left the room. When he came back, he was relaxed, for whatever reason, and started talking with the patient quite actively about school and sports. The teenager responded enthusiastically. I observed how engaged they were in the conversation (I will say more about engagement later). After a few moments, the student looked at his watch and said, *"Well, we better get back to the interview."* Together, and as before, the student stiffened up and again took out his list while the teenager looked down. This story illustrates that communication is a natural behavior, and it happened after the phone call when the medical interview was not occurring. Then the student's attempt to do the interview set up nonverbal obstacles that interfered with the communication process. This experience became a teaching moment for the student.

Nonverbal communication pre-dates the development of language and establishes a sense of connection. Gestures, physical distance/closeness, and nonverbal signals always were and still are the most genuine and immutable forms of communication. Nonverbal images are encoded in the most primitive areas of the brain and connect to emotional centers that are not readily modifiable by conscious intent. Experts in nonverbal communication, including experienced clinicians and psychologists, not to mention FBI agents and magicians, know that people can deceive and mislead with their words but not by their nonverbal communication. Nonverbal communication also carries emotion, and when communication is favorable, it creates trustworthiness, connection, and truth. In the 1970s, psychologists began studying dyadic interactions in singles bars. They found that the nonverbal behavior of bodily synchrony was associated with a sense of connection. Couples who automatically mimicked each other nonverbally in synchrony were emotionally engaged. They leaned the same way or together crossed or uncrossed their legs.

I have often observed a patient gently stroke down on the upper back part of the cheekbone (zygomaticus) when discussing a loss or a sad memory. Yes, symbolically, that is wiping a tear; it is usually unconscious and universal. When I applied for training programs, I noted during my interview that I better say something more satisfying if the interviewer crossed their arms, or it might not go well.

My mentor, George Engel, first taught me the gesture of helplessness. We have all observed it, and we register our understanding of the feelings it generates, but we may not always articulate what it means. The person is sitting in the chair, and you ask, *"How was your day?"* They discuss a problematic series of events, perhaps not meeting deadlines or getting into an argument with the boss. Concurrently, they raise one or both hands, palms facing inward, and then suddenly drop them, as if by gravity. That would be a signal for me to say empathically, *"You must have felt helpless."* In most cases, the patients would acknowledge my comment. This nonverbal gesture validates the feelings surrounding the person's verbal report of the day's experience. The helplessness gesture is rooted in childhood: if you were 3 years old, where would you gesture for help? But what if you raised your hands and there was no help? The second part of the gesture is to let gravity lower the hands, which symbolizes the non-availability of help. These are universal gestures that occur across all cultures.

These are examples to underscore the value of observing, understanding, and applying nonverbal communication in the clinical setting. Patients and doctors can assess each other's level of engagement and find ways to improve the interaction; they can learn from each other.

So, let's go to the clinical situation. Take a moment to look at Figure 26 of a doctor and a patient. What do you see, without hearing the words? How do you feel the visit is going?

I use this photo in lectures to illustrate a nonverbal communication technique known as engagement. Yes, people get engaged to marry, but in health care, engagement means an interaction or connection between the patient and the doctor who are working together toward common goals in the plan of care.

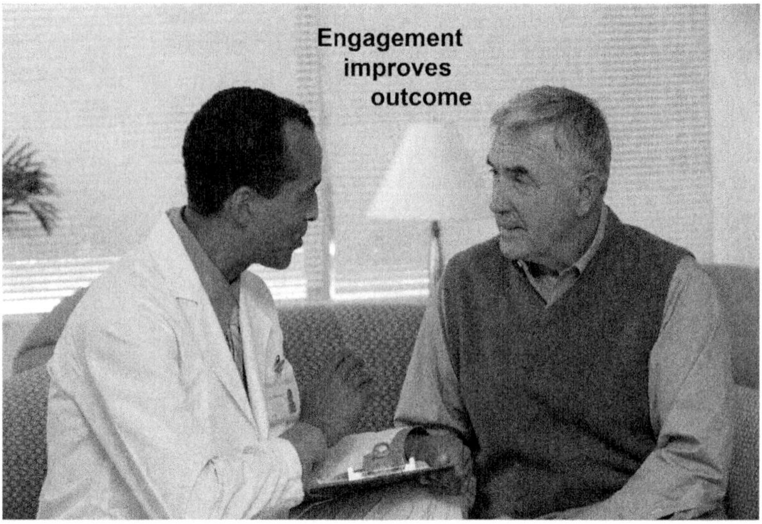


**Figure 26.** Nonverbal features of engagement

As shown in the photo, engagement is characterized by:

- Good eye contact
- Affirmative nods and gestures
- A gentle tone of voice
- Close interpersonal distance
- A partner-like relationship

Below is another, more detailed cartoon of nonverbal communication that is (1) ineffective and (2) effective (see Figure 27). Again, with no words spoken, if you were the patient, how would you feel? Now you know why.

Engagement is a form of nonverbal communication that is associated with higher degrees of patient satisfaction, a sense of connection, adherence to treatment, and even improved clinical outcomes.[58] To see a demonstration of these nonverbal communication methods go to **https://romedross.video/Q_A_NonverbComm**.

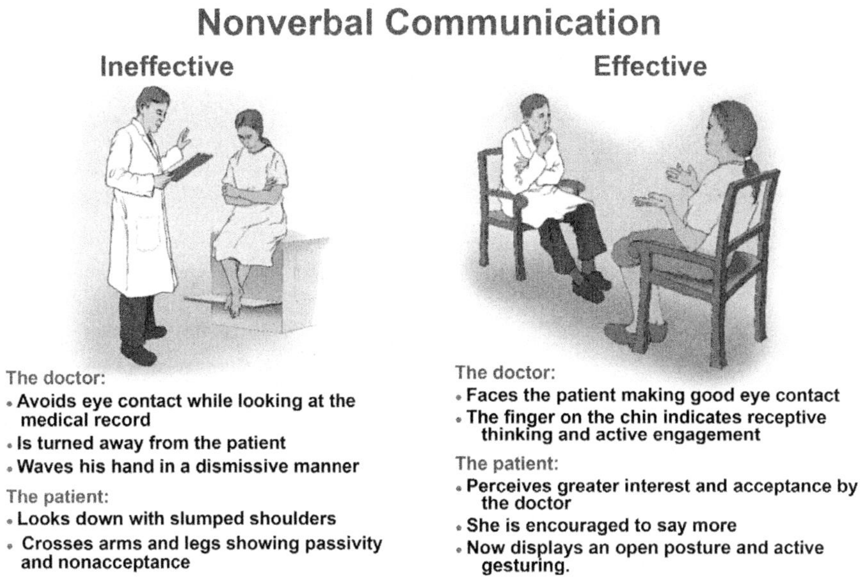


**Figure 27.** Ineffective and effective nonverbal communication. From Ruddy J. From pretending to truly being OK: A journey from illness to health with postinfection irritable bowel syndrome. Gastroenterology 2018;155:1666–1669.

Now we can summarize this information. Table 3, below, presents a detailed list of verbal and nonverbal behaviors on the part of the doctor that promote or hinder the patient-doctor relationship.

*Table 3. Verbal and Nonverbal Behaviors Affecting Communication*[50]

| BEHAVIOR | FACILITATES | INHIBITS |
|---|---|---|
| **Nonverbal** | | |
| Clinical environment | Private, comfortable | Noisy, physical barriers |
| Eye contact | Frequent | Infrequent or constant |
| Listening | Active listening—questions relate to what patient says | Distracted or preoccupied (e.g. typing) |
| Body posture | Direct, open, relaxed | Body turned, arms folded, |
| Head nodding | Well timed | Infrequent, excessive |
| Body proximity | Close enough to touch | Too close or too distant |
| Facial expression | Shows interest and understanding | Preoccupation, boredom, disapproval |
| Voice | Gentle tone | Harsh, rushed |
| Touching | Helpful if well timed and used to communicate empathy | Insincere if inappropriate or not properly timed |
| Synchrony (arms, legs) | Concordant | Discordant |

*continues*

| BEHAVIOR | FACILITATES | INHIBITS |
|---|---|---|
| **Verbal** | | |
| Question forms | Open-ended to generate hypotheses | Rigid or stereotyped style |
| | Closed-ended to test hypotheses | Multiple choice or leading questions ("You didn't... did you?) |
| | Use of patient's words | Use of unfamiliar words or jargon |
| | Facilitates patient discussion by "echoing" or affirmative gestures | Interruptions, undue control of conversation |
| | Uses summarizing statements | Not done |
| Question/Interview style | Nonjudgmental | Judgmental |
| | Follows lead of patient's prior comments (patient centered) | Follows own preset agenda or style |
| | Use of a narrative thread | Unorganized questioning |
| | Appropriate use of silence | Interruptions or too much silence |
| | Appropriate reassurance and encouragement | Premature or unwarranted reassurance or encouragement |
| | Communicates empathy | Not provided or not sincere |
| Recommendations | Elicits feedback and negotiates | No feedback, states views directly |
| Asks/Provides medical information | As appropriate to the clinical issues | Too many biomedical questions and too detailed information |
| Asks/Provides psycho-social information | Elicits in a sensitive and non-threatening manner | Ignores psychosocial data or asks intrusive or probing questions |
| Humor | When appropriate and facili-tative | None or inappropriate humor |

Now that we have discussed the communication skills that build on the PDR, have a look at the following video and see how many of these elements you can recognize: http://bit.ly/2H7MHb3.

## *The Patient's Role*[39]

Within this partnership, your responsibility is to work with your doctor to make all the right things happen that we've addressed to achieve positive outcomes. The value of a partnership is that no one person is entirely responsible. The wins and losses are shared and discussed together. With that in mind, you need to have realistic expectations of your doctor, who has no "magic wand" for diagnosing and treating chronic illness. The doctor has scientific knowledge, but they may need some time to make a confident diagnosis and ensure that they are not overlooking other factors. Similarly, with treatment, as we've discussed, you are responsible for appraising the information to make a proper treatment decision. The following guidelines help you to establish a good PDR and to participate in the management of your illness.

### *Starting and conducting the visit*

- **Bring a family member or friend if you want.** They can provide support, offer additional questions, and help you remember important things after the appointment.
- **Be clear and concise on the goals of the visit.** Tell the doctor why you are seeking their help and what your expectations are.
- **Ask the right questions.** Think about what you want to ask before you show up for your appointment. Having a brief list of issues or questions can help you to organize your thoughts—just be aware that long lists can be distracting and may interfere with good communication. Also, remember that the list is to help you to communicate more effectively—not as a replacement—so don't give it to your doctor.
- **Express your thoughts, feelings, and concerns.** Your thoughts, feelings, and concerns are valid and must address them for you to feel confident to participate in your diagnosis and treatment. There are no "dumb" questions. Your doctor can't speak to your worries if they don't know what they are.
- **Be honest.** Explain your perspective on your symptoms (onset, frequency, duration, impact on your quality of life). Don't just tell the doctor what you think they want to hear.
- **Share difficult issues (such as loss, grief, abuse).** This can be especially difficult and scary, and so much depends on your comfort level and sense of trust in the doctor. You might start slowly by recalling a distressing event: "*Things were pretty difficult back then. . . .* " If you see the doctor listening and engaging, and even encouraging you to go on, it's safe to do so. You may then begin a dialog that could potentially be healing. However, if the doctor seems distracted or changes the topic, it's best to save it for another time. . . .

### *Negotiating diagnosis and treatment*

- **Be an assertive and confident partner.** As discussed, patient-centered care requires your participation. You work with the doctor on setting the goals for care, and selecting diagnostic approaches and treatments. Be honest in responding to the doctor's questions. Ask for clarification or further explanation when you need it and state any concerns. The final decision is yours, but the doctor must provide the knowledge to guide you in your decisions.
- **Work with the doctor to customize a treatment plan that works best for you.** Treatment plans can involve a multi-tiered approach such as diet, exercise, medication, and even the addition of brain-gut psychological therapies such as mindfulness, CBT, or gut-directed hypnotherapy to manage chronic pain. These choices may be recommended sequentially or in combination. You and the doctor need to consider what the next treatment options are if the first sequence doesn't work. To help in treatment planning, you need to know how each treatment works, the side effects, effectiveness, and how long it will take. Then before you proceed with any treatment—you need to be honest in your views about the treatment options. It is essential to feel good about engaging in the management plan.
- **Determine your doctor's commitment to work with you.** With a chronic illness like DGBI, you will need a doctor to provide ongoing care. Therefore, it is reasonable for you to ask, during your first visit, if your doctor is able and willing to work with you long term. If a doctor indicates that they are committed to long-term care in a partnership with you and does not maintain this level of commitment, the relationship will be weak. You have the right to address this observation with your doctor or go elsewhere.
- **Be aware of your rights in the healthcare process.** Patients can receive inadequate care when doctors are dismissive or stigmatizing. These patients are at risk of suffering in silence or going from doctor to doctor, trying to find answers, and each encounter produces more frustration. You have the right to be treated with respect and to ask questions and voice objections or opinions. You also have the right to seek a second opinion, without feeling guilt or shame. Finally, you have the right to say no to treatment.

### *What if there are problems during the visit with your doctor?*

Most doctors are well-intentioned, committed to helping their patients, willing to learn, and eager to provide the best of care. This section will address the infrequent occasions when a medical visit does not go well. I hear many patients complaining about their previous doctor being inept or mistreating them. There may be some truth to that in some cases, but it does take two to tango. A few years ago, I was conducting a workshop with a colleague to help patients improve communication with their doctors. On stage, we demonstrated a medical visit and trained the simulated doctor to perform his role reasonably well. Then we prepared the simulated patient to demonstrate ineffective behaviors: answering their cell phone, not being aware of their medication, not actively listening, cutting into the doctor's statements, and so on. When we asked the audience for their feedback, we were surprised to hear that most of their comments were criticisms about the doctor's performance. The group discussion that followed taught us that many of the patients had become so emotionally distraught from their negative personal experiences with their doctors that they had become blind to what they may or may not have done that contributed to the problematic interaction. The group then learned that there are methods they can use to reshape the communication with their doctor when it doesn't go well, and which increases their degree of control. That was an empowering moment for the group.

Listed below are some ineffective scenarios that may occur during the doctor visit and some suggestions for what you can do to improve them. While it may seem strange that we are teaching patients how to give feedback to their doctors, that kind of communication and feedback are the heart of patient-centered care. It's a two-way process, and your role is to contribute to the partnership. When providing feedback, it is essential to comment on your experience, rather than being critical of the doctor's behavior.

**The doctor appears rushed.** This may be the most common complaint and is often due to many understandable factors these days: the visit started late, the doctor is being interrupted by the nurse or getting urgent messages, completing the electronic medical record (EMR) is taking up a lot of time, and so on. We may presume that the doctor being rushed relates to their stress about being unable to do their proper job of attending to the visit. So, a simple comment such as: *"I'm sorry you have so many diversions. It's okay; please take your time."* This comment lets the doctor know that you understand the dilemma and are trying to help.

Sometimes, however, rushed behavior reflects more challenging issues: a fixed and ineffective communication style; inadequate training in communication skills; negative, dualism-based views toward working with patients who have a DGBI; having a terrible day; or just not wanting to be in the clinic at all. To address this, the patient may start with an inquiry, *"It seems a lot is going on. Is there anything I can do to help?"* The response to this can be telling. If the question helps to refocus the doctor's behavior, their response might be: *"I'm sorry, yes, it's a bad day..."* and the conduct of the visit may improve. If the answer does not address your question or the behavior continues, you might say after a few more minutes: *"I don't feel like I'm able to talk about my problems very well. Is there anything we can do to improve that?"* If at this point, the visit doesn't improve, a final response would be: *"I'm not feeling satisfied with the way the visit is going. Is there some reason for that?"* If the doctor bypasses the comment or doesn't reflect any concerns, the patient needs to decide whether to accept the visit as a lousy one for the day or consider future options for care.

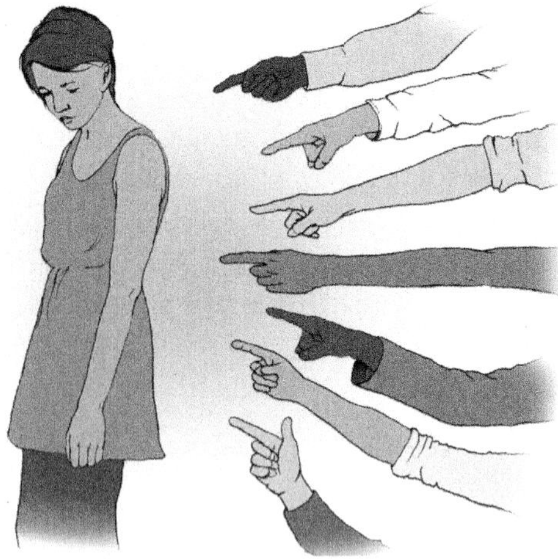

Figure 28. Stigma

**The doctor seems dismissive or stigmatizing (see Figure 28).** Negative comments from the doctor can be hurtful. If the doctor says: *"The tests are negative. I believe your problem is due to stress. You work and also have three children, so you need to relax."* The doctor's comments may represent not understanding the patient's responsibilities, an ineffective attempt to be empathic, or a lack of knowledge of what to do. Even worse, they may be pejorative.

When these statements are made, the doctor may naively not be anticipating the impact on the patient, and needs to be educated.

The patient needs to determine if the doctor's comments truly reflect these negative behaviors or are being misinterpreted. Here, questioning for clarification is in order: *"Doctor, I may be under stress, but I didn't hear from you my medical diagnosis. I also don't understand your plan for how to manage this. Can you clarify this?"* The response can provide some insight into the doctor's understanding and perception of the problem and can help guide the next step. If you hear a change in the response that feels more satisfying, the visit can continue. If, however, the doctor's comments are unchanged, you might say: *"I'm sorry, but what you are saying makes me feel like it's my fault. I need to understand my diagnosis and how we are going to treat it."* At this point, if the doctor seems defensive or argumentative, it might be a message to reconsider your choice of doctors.

**The doctor seems unknowledgeable.** In some cases, the doctor may not be familiar with the diagnostic approach for DGBI. Here, the doctor orders many tests looking for a structural abnormality—and if they are negative, continues to do so. However, with DGBI, the knowledgeable doctor makes the diagnosis using Rome criteria and does some screening studies to exclude other diseases. If these are negative, the doctor can then convey confidence in the diagnosis and focus on management. A few doctors who are not familiar with DGBI may "hang their hat" on a diagnosis that gives biological credibility but is inconsistent with the clinical findings. Many patients come to me with inaccurate or inconclusive diagnoses of small intestinal bacterial overgrowth (SIBO), gastroparesis, Lyme disease, median arcuate ligament syndrome (MALS), parasitic infection, mast cell disease, and many more. In these situations, their former doctor may have felt more comfortable using a seemingly credible label rather than communicate uncertainty. In so doing, however, they were either not knowledgeable of the correct diagnosis and proper treatment or bypassed the real diagnosis. Finally, a few doctors may not believe in DGBI and merely treat the symptoms without a clear understanding of the pathophysiology to guide the management. For all these situations, the patient can request further information. *"Doctor, can you give me some additional information to help me understand what I have and what my treatment options will be?"* The doctor does not need to be a world expert; what is important is for them to be open to learning more. So if it appears that they are uncertain about a topic or any question you ask, their best response would be: *"I don't know that, but I'll check into that and get back to you."*

If you continue to feel dissatisfied in the care you are receiving, keep in mind that the field of neurogastroenterology—which encompasses motility disorders and disorders of gut-brain interaction—is growing. Many doctors in this field are at major medical centers or large clinics. The Rome Foundation (**www.theromefoundation.org**) has a membership of many gastroenterologists who dedicate themselves to treating patients with these disorders. Also, Appendix B of this book lists clinical resources where patients with DGBI can be evaluated and treated.

### *Moving forward after the visit*

**Address expectations and set realistic goals.** Once you have a diagnosis and treatment plan, your role is to set realistic management goals to move toward recovery. Sometimes this means resetting priorities. For example, if symptoms kept you from going to your child's sporting events, make that a new goal to achieve by following recommendations for rest, diet, medication, and stress reduction. This might mean saying *no* to other things so that you can prioritize your health and family. It is within your power and control to say *no*, for the sake of your health, to what is not essential.

**Find your new life.** Once you have established a positive relationship with your doctor and are managing your health as a team, try to focus on other key areas of your life that bring you meaning and joy. Instead of focusing on what you cannot do, focus on what you *can* do to bring back control and normalcy.

**Remember that you are not alone.** Other patients share your illness and burden. Your doctor is your partner in managing this with you. Family and friends may also want to help. There *is* hope for you to move forward and maintain your health long term, and not alone.

## PART 4

# What the Doctor Is Doing, or Should Be Doing

*"Care more particularly to the individual patient than for the special features of the disease."*
—Sir William Osler, 1849–1919, Albany Med Ass 1899;20:307–309

This section has a dual purpose. The first is for you, as the patient, to understand what the doctor is doing or should be doing, and why. We are looking to make more transparent the clinical behaviors that doctors use to make a diagnosis or to treat, so you know what to expect. This information may also help you to understand when things are not going as well as they should. Also, this part is for doctors to learn how to best approach the care of patients with DGBI. The field of neurogastroenterology (i.e., the DGBI), as a subsection of gastroenterology, is relatively new in concept, diagnosis, and treatment. Many doctors in primary care or even gastroenterology who are not familiar with neurogastroenterological concepts may, therefore, benefit from seeing how we recommend the application of this new knowledge.

### Diagnosis

To begin with, doctors should be saying "Disorders of Gut-Brain Interaction" (DGBI). This new term moves us away from the dualistic "Functional GI Disorder" model (**https://romedross.video/Q_A_fgid_dgbi**); it legitimizes the diagnosis and provides a scientific basis to explain and characterize these symptoms and disorders.

Next, doctors should apply the Rome IV symptom-based criteria and exclude, cost-effectively, other specific conditions having similar clinical presentations. This means conducting a proper physical examination, including a rectal examination,[59] ordering appropriate laboratory tests, and, when needed, x-ray or endoscopic imaging. These tests help to identify medical diagnoses that have similar symptoms but will require different, more specific treatments. For example, abdominal pain and diarrhea are features of IBS-D but also occur with celiac disease, in which treatment requires dietary gluten restriction; or Crohn's disease, which is treated with anti-inflammatory or immunosuppressive therapies. Doctors use their wisdom—the combination of their knowledge, experience, and sound judgment—to discern when diagnostic procedures are needed and when they should be avoided, particularly if unnecessary and costly.[1] For example, a young patient returning from a vacation in a tropical country with a day or two of abdominal cramps and diarrhea may have a stool test to find an infection or just receive symptomatic treatment; the doctor will wait to see if the symptoms resolve.

Conversely, an older patient with a more extended period of pain and diarrhea who is losing weight because the pain prevents him from eating will require many more tests, including CT scan or endoscopy. Also, the type of symptoms helps to determine the studies. Nausea and vomiting would lead to doing an upper endoscopy, while lower abdominal pain may lead to blood tests, colonoscopy, and possibly a CT scan.

Skilled doctors also consider many other factors. For example, regardless of the possible diagnosis, a patient over 50 should get a colonoscopy to screen for colon cancer. The wise doctor will select more studies when a patient's symptoms are new or have recently changed in their quality or severity, or if there are no previous diagnostic studies. They will order the appropriate tests when they find alarm signs or "red flags" that may point to another diagnosis. Alarm signs may include weight loss, anemia, blood in the stool, a family history of inflammatory bowel disease or cancer, or an abnormal physical examination or laboratory studies. The Rome Foundation has developed a set of guidelines called algorithms that doctors can use to guide them through what may be, at times, a complex diagnostic process:[60] **https://romedross.video/2Y7yEwT**. Figure 29 demonstrates the evaluation pathway for patients presenting with abdominal pain and bowel difficulties.[60] Here is a video demonstration using the diagnostic algorithm via the Rome Foundation's GI Genius intelligent software: **https://romedross.video/Q_ADiagnosingGIGenius**.

It's also important to know that when patients with chronic illness are in pain and distress, they may urgently request diagnostic procedures to "*find out what's wrong*." Inexperienced doctors adhering to the dualistic model feel helpless when this happens because they don't understand the problem and may feel compelled to order tests out of concern that something is being missed. The term "furor medicus"[61] was coined decades ago to reflect the vicious cycle of test-ordering and even unwarranted surgery that ensues from this emotional response. Nowadays, we have the science of the biopsychosocial and brain-gut models and validated diagnostic criteria to define DGBI. Therefore, we can reverse this cycle of seeking studies out of uncertainty. Providing the knowledge to legitimize the DGBI as bona fide disorders, offering proper education and reassurance, and clarifying that the focus is not on further testing but on proper management through patient-centered care, reverses the vicious cycle and satisfies the patient.

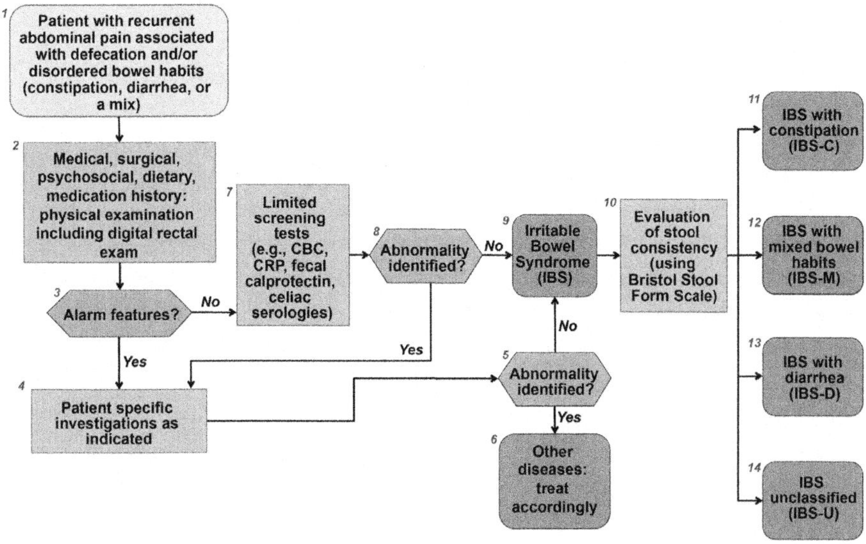


**Figure 29.** A diagnostic algorithm for a patient presenting with abdominal pain and disordered bowel habits. The Rome Foundation developed pathways for all the DGBI.[60] Purple represents a diagnosis. Gold represents a decision path with "yes" and "no" exit paths. Green directs toward a diagnostic test or therapeutic action. From Mearin F, Bowel Disorders, In: Kellow J, Drossman DA, Chang L, et al: Rome IV Diagnostic Algorithms for Common GI Symptoms. 2016, 3rd ed. Raleigh (NC) Rome Foundation.

## Treatment

Treatment is based on a biopsychosocial understanding of illness related to brain-gut axis dysregulation. The DGBI is defined by any of the following: motility disturbance, visceral hypersensitivity, altered mucosal and immune function, altered gut microbiota, and altered central nervous system processing.[3] Therefore, patients meeting Rome IV criteria for a DGBI may have any combination of these factors producing varied symptom features. For example, a patient with IBS may have bloating related to ingesting large amounts of fermentable oligo-, di-, or mono-saccharides, and polyols (FODMAPs); pain and diarrhea related to visceral hypersensitivity; altered mucosal immune functioning as a result of a previous bacterial infection (post-infection IBS); or anxiety and pain due to central pain dysregulation from post-traumatic stress disorder following sexual or physical trauma. Since the clinical profile and severity may change over time, the discerning doctor needs to identify which of these factors alone, or in combination, are targets for treatment. When initiating treatment, there are several principles to consider.

## The Symptom Profile

The type of symptoms, their location, and the physiological determinants will all influence treatment. Therefore, constipation symptoms or IBS-C may be treated by secretagogues like Linzess (linaclotide), Trulance (plecanatide), or Amitiza (lubiprostone), which increase fluid secretion by activating intestinal ion channels; or a prokinetic agent such as Zelnorm (tegaserod) or Motegrity (prucalopride), which increase motility by activating 5-hydroxytryptamine (5-HT) receptors. In contrast, for IBS-D, an antibiotic like Xifaxan (rifaximin) may be useful because it may restore a better microbiome. In addition, a serotonergic (5HT3) receptor antagonist like Lotronex (alosetron) or Zofran (ondansetron), or even a mixed opioid-receptor medication like Viberzi (eluxadoline) will treat the pain and diarrhea by altering gut neurotransmitters and receptors. However, if the abdominal pain is severe, treatment might also include a central neuromodulator; if the pain is localized to the rectum (e.g., Levator Ani Syndrome), anorectal biofeedback may be used. The doctor needs to identify the symptom profile (i.e., which symptom features are dominant), and from that, determine which treatment(s) are most likely to lead to improvement.

## Psychosocial Features

The brain-gut axis is the basis for a bidirectional relationship in which gastrointestinal symptoms influence the psychosocial state, and vice versa, as we fully discussed in Part 1. The doctor must emphasize that chronic pain, nausea, or vomiting can lead to anxiety or depression, as modified by early experiences, coping, and social and family influences. Conversely, psychosocial difficulties, including comorbid anxiety, depression, a significant loss, or a history of sexual or physical trauma, influence pain threshold and gastrointestinal motility. By clarifying that there is no one cause, but a combination of factors, the doctor can minimize the patient's perception of stigma, which is relating the cause of their symptoms to stress or psychiatric disease.

This understanding justifies the use of brain-gut behavioral therapies such as cognitive-behavioral therapy, gut-directed hypnotherapy, and mindfulness meditation.[27, 62] Patient motivation to engage in these treatments predicts success.[27] The best candidates for brain-gut behavioral therapies understand the nature of gut-brain disorders, are open to behavioral change to alleviate symptoms, can make connections between times of stress and anxiety and symptoms, and have the time to participate in the treatment. Patients with severe psychopathology or personality disorder, who have little insight into the gut-brain interaction, who primarily focus on a "cure," or who are unable or unwilling to commit to treatment, are unlikely to benefit.

## Symptom Severity

Severity is a biopsychosocial composite of patient-reported gastrointestinal and extra-intestinal symptoms, the degree of pain, disability, psychosocial impairments, illness-related perceptions and behaviors, and health-related quality of life.[63] Severity plays a significant role in selecting treatments. For example, a patient with infrequent, low-grade abdominal pain, and no other symptoms or psychological distress who is unlikely to go to the doctor would be classified as mild, and not treated. Conversely, a patient having severe abdominal pain, along with fibromyalgia and migraine headaches, who is unable to work, depressed, and frequently seeks health care—or needs hospitalization—would be considered severe and treated with behavioral and multiple medical treatments. Table 4 (page 130) provides guidelines developed by a Rome Foundation working team and modified to help categorize severity for DGBI.[63] What follows is the categorization of patients with mild, moderate, and severe symptoms. This approach allows doctors to optimize the treatment.[15]

**Mild symptoms.** Patients with mild or infrequent symptoms comprise about 40% of patients, are seen more in primary care than in gastroenterology practices, and do not have significant impairment in function or psychological distress. Their symptoms often relate to gastrointestinal dysfunction (i.e., vomiting, diarrhea, constipation), and their pain is mild and without other physical symptoms. Patients with mild symptoms do not usually have other psychiatric diagnoses, and their quality of life is good. Still, they may report concerns about how their symptoms affect their lives and say that a stressful event may worsen their symptoms. These patients do not make frequent medical visits and usually maintain healthy activity levels without restriction. In these cases, treatment focuses on:

*Education.* The doctor should indicate that DGBI are real disorders in which the gastrointestinal system is overly responsive to a variety of stimuli, such as food, hormonal changes, medication, and stress. Pain can result from spasm or stretching of the gut, or a sensitive gut, and can be experienced anywhere in the abdomen. It can also be associated with other effects on gastrointestinal function, leading to symptoms such as pain, nausea, vomiting, and diarrhea. Physiological and psychological factors interact to produce symptoms.

*Reassurance.* The doctor should offer appropriate reassurance based on the patient's concerns. Reassurance should be based on scientific data and not presented in a superficial manner. In general, the doctor should indicate their availability if new or different symptoms arise.

*Diet and medication.* Offending dietary substances (e.g., lactose, FODMAPs, caffeine, fatty foods, alcohol) and medicines that adversely affect symptoms should be identified and reduced or eliminated.

**Moderate symptoms.** About 30–35% of patients seen in primary or secondary care report moderate symptoms, with intermittent disruptions in daily activities such as missing social functions, work, or school. They may identify a close relationship between symptoms and inciting events such as dietary indiscretion, travel, or distressing experiences. Their symptoms, including abdominal pain, are moderate, and they may be more psychologically distressed than patients with mild symptoms. Several other medical or psychological difficulties may co-exist, and these patients may lose time from work or need to curtail usual functioning. For this group, we recommend additional treatments:

*Symptom monitoring.* The patient can keep a symptom diary for 1–2 weeks to record the time, severity, and presence of associated factors. This will help to identify inciting factors, such as dietary indiscretions or specific stressors, not previously considered. The physician can then review possible nutritional, lifestyle, or behavioral influences with the patient. A diary can encourage the patient's participation in treatment and, as symptoms improve, increase their sense of control over the illness.

*Pharmacotherapy directed at specific symptoms.* Symptom episodes that are more frequent, long-lasting, or distressing, or that impair daily function, usually require prescription medications. The choice of medication depends upon the predominant symptoms, as described above. In general, prescription medications are ancillary to dietary or lifestyle modifications for mild chronic symptoms. They are used during periods of acute symptom exacerbation, or regularly for moderate or severe symptoms.

*Brain-gut behavioral treatments.* These types of psychological treatments may be considered for motivated patients with moderate to severe GI symptoms and pain. The treatments are more helpful if the patient can associate symptoms with stressors. They include cognitive behavior therapy, relaxation, hypnosis, mindfulness, and combination treatments, help to reduce anxiety levels, encourage health-promoting behaviors, and give the patient greater responsibility and control in their treatment and in potentially improving their pain tolerance.

**Severe symptoms.** About 20–25% of patients with DGBI most often seen in referral practices have severe symptoms, and a smaller proportion has very severe unremitting symptoms. These patients, like Ms. Byers in the introduction of this book, also have associated psychosocial difficulties, including anxiety, depression, illness anxiety, somatic symptoms disorder, or personality disturbance, along with chronically impaired daily functioning. About 10% or more have a work disability. There may be a history of significant loss or abuse, poor social networks or coping skills, and "catastrophic" thinking. Perhaps in response to experiences in the healthcare system, they may feel stigmatized for their condition and deny or refuse to consider a role for psychosocial factors in their illness. As a result, they may be unwilling to engage in the psychological or psychopharmacological treatment. They will often continue to seek diagnostic studies to legitimize their complaints and select pharmacological treatments directed at the gut. For this group, we recommend additional treatment options:

*The doctor's approach.* These patients need an ongoing relationship with a doctor (gastroenterologist, advanced practice provider, or primary care doctor) who provides psychosocial support through brief ongoing visits. Patients with severe symptoms don't want to be abandoned, and their relationship with the doctor helps them to maintain a sense of hope. In general, the doctor should: (a) perform diagnostic and therapeutic measures based on objective findings, rather than as a response to patient demands; (b) set realistic treatment goals, such as improved quality of life, rather than complete pain relief or cure; (c) shift the responsibility for treatment to the patient by giving therapeutic options; (d) change the focus of care from treating the disease to adjusting to and managing chronic illness; and e) maintain continuity of care.

*Central neuromodulator treatment.* If pain is a dominant feature, tricyclic antidepressants (TCAs) such as Norpramin (desipramine) or Elavil (amitriptyline) and the serotonin-norepinephrine reuptake inhibitors (SNRIs) such as Cymbalta (duloxetine) control the pain via central analgesia. It may also relieve associated psychological distress. The selective serotonin reuptake inhibitors (SSRIs), such as Celexa (citalopram) or Prozac (fluoxetine), may have an ancillary role; they are less useful for pain due to the lack of noradrenergic effect but can help reduce anxiety and associated depression. Central neuromodulators should help patients with chronic pain and impaired daily functioning, concurrent symptoms of major or atypical depression, symptom anxiety, or panic attacks. Even without depressive symptoms, these agents may help when the pain is dominant and consuming. An inadequate clinical response may be due to insufficient dose or failure to adjust the dosage based on the therapeutic response or side effects. Combination treatment (augmentation) is prescribed if a single medication is not helpful or if there are side effects. Further detail on the use of central neuromodulators is available elsewhere.[25]

*Brain-gut behavioral treatments.* These psychological treatments may also be helpful for patients having severe GI symptoms. Usually, central neuromodulators are used concurrently with these treatments. The doctor needs to ensure that the patient understands the potential value of these treatments and is motivated to engage in the care process. My research has shown that the strongest predictors of improvement with cognitive-behavioral therapy include: the patient's belief that they will benefit, their motivation to commit to the treatment, and their relationship with the therapist. The types of treatments are similar to those seen with moderate symptoms. However, they may also include dialectical behavior therapy (DBT), which may be better suited to patients with more severe psychological distress who require help with emotional regulation, adjusting to stress, and improving interpersonal relationships. Some studies suggest that patients with PTSD or early trauma may benefit from Eye Movement Desensitization and Reprocessing Training (EMDR), but this technique still requires further validation.

*Neurogastroenterology pain treatment center referral.* There are several GI programs and pain treatment centers that provide a multidisciplinary approach to DGBI management. See Appendix B. In these instances, the team approach is directed toward pain management, improved coping skills, and overall rehabilitation of patients who have become disabled. See the appendix for a list of resources.

Table 4 represents the parameters we consider in determining symptom severity.

*Table 4. Clinical Profile for Severity in Disorders of Gut-Brain Interaction*[63, 64]

| Clinical Feature | Mild | Moderate | Severe |
|---|---|---|---|
| Estimated prevalence | 40% | 35% | 25% |
| Symptom severity | Low | Medium | High |
| Physiological factors | Primarily gastrointestinal dysfunction | Gastrointestinal dysfunction and CNS pain dysregulation | Primarily CNS pain dysregulation |
| Psychosocial difficulties | None or mild psychological distress | Moderate psychological distress | Severe psychological distress, catastrophizing, abuse history |
| Abdominal pain | Mild, intermittent | Moderate, frequent | Severe, very frequent, or constant |
| Number of extra-intestinal symptoms | Low (1–3) | Medium (4–6) | High (7 or more) |
| Health-related quality of life | Good | Fair | Poor |
| Frequency of doctor visits | 0–1 time per year | 2–4 times per year | 5 or more times per year |
| Activity restriction | Occasional (0–15 days) | More often (15–50 days) | Frequent or constant (more than 50 days) |
| Work disability | <5% | 6–10% | 11% or greater |

Figure 30 demonstrates the relationship of brain-gut influences on the continuum of DGBI, from mild to severe, and their possible treatments. The triangle shows the relative frequency of these disorders. Patients having mild symptoms are the most frequent and comprise most of the size of the triangle; patients with more severe symptoms are less frequent, as shown on the right (see Table 4). The top of the figure shows the influences on symptom severity, which are primarily bowel-

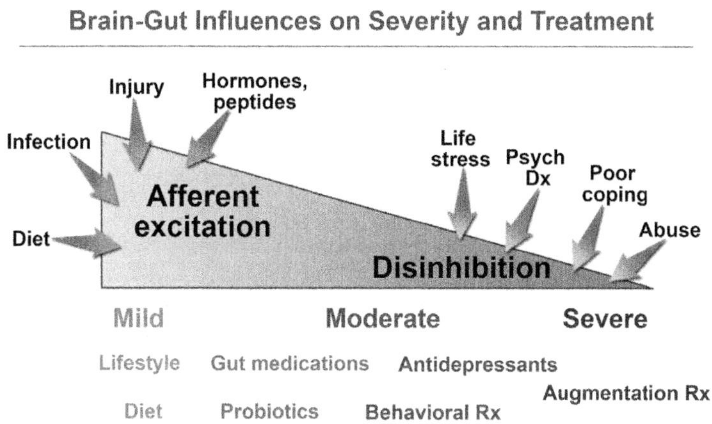


**Figure 30.** The continuum of severity for DGBI, their influences, and treatment. Afferent excitation relates to the nerve signals coming from the gut (visceral hypersensitivity). Disinhibition refers to the brain's inability to send nerve signals down the gut-brain axis to block pain coming up to the brain. See text above for further details.

related on the left, as influenced by dietary indiscretion, dysmotility, infection, etc. However, the right side shows how the central nervous system (CNS) influences symptoms when more severe, and relates to psychosocial distress affecting brain regulation of symptoms. Finally, at the bottom, we see that the kinds of treatments to be considered relate to the degree of severity. With mild illness, diet and lifestyle modifications would be helpful; with more severe symptoms, we use neuromodulators and behavioral interventions.

In summary, the treatment of DGBI requires a multimodal approach that takes the nature of symptoms into account, as well as their severity, the presence of associated psychosocial difficulties that we call comorbidities, and how they impact each other. The Rome Foundation has developed the Multidimensional Clinical Profile (MDCP), which takes these considerations into account to help the doctor provide care that is targeted to the personal needs of the patient.[65]

These are the five components of this Multidimensional Clinical (MDCP) Profile:

A. Categorical diagnosis (these are the symptom-based criteria)
B. Clinical modifier (e.g., IBS-C, IBS-D, IBS-M, post-infection etiology, FODMAP sensitivity)
C. Impact (mild, moderate, severe)
D. Psychosocial modifier (e.g., psychological diagnosis, loss, trauma history)
E. Physiological dysfunction and biomarkers (when available)

The MDCP book, which lays this information in more detail using clinical case reports, is available through the Rome Foundation: **https://romedross.video/MDCP**.

## Fourteen Tips to Improve Patient-Doctor Communication

In Part 3, we discussed in some detail the methods of communication to optimize the patient-doctor relationship (PDR). Studies show that the PDR improves patient and doctor satisfaction, adherence to treatment, symptom reduction, and other health outcomes.[1, 50] Below is a summary of recommendations the doctor can use in patient care.

1. **Seek to improve patient satisfaction and engagement.** Patient satisfaction relates to their perception of the doctor's humaneness, technical competence, interest in psychosocial factors, and provision of relevant medical information. Engagement relies on nonverbal communication: good eye contact, affirmative nods, gentle tone of voice, close interpersonal distance, and creation of a partner-like interaction. It helps to check in with the patient with a question like "*How are these visits going for you?*" This can yield valuable feedback on the quality of the interaction and the degree of patient satisfaction.

2. **Obtain the history through a nondirective, nonjudgmental, patient-centered interview.** This involves active listening, as well as asking questions based on the patient's thoughts, feelings, and experiences rather than using a personal or preset agenda of items. The interview can begin with: "*It's very nice to meet you, . . . how can I help?*" This sets the stage for the patient to know you are interested and available.

3. **Determine the immediate reason for the patient's visit.** The doctor can ask: "*What led you to see me at this time?*" and evaluate the patient's verbal and nonverbal responses. Consider the following possibilities:
   a. new or exacerbating factors (dietary change, concurrent medical disorder, side effects of new medication)
   b. personal concern about a serious disease (e.g., recent family death)
   c. personal or family stressors (e.g., current or a past anniversary of a death or other significant loss, abuse event or history)
   d. worsening or development of psychiatric comorbidity (depression, anxiety)
   e. impairment in daily function (recent inability to work or socialize)
   f. a "hidden agenda," such as narcotic or laxative abuse, pending litigation, or disability claims.

4. **Conduct a careful physical examination and cost-efficient investigation.** A well-conducted physical examination has therapeutic value.[47]

5. **Determine what the patient understands of the illness and what their concerns are.** Questions to ask include: "*What do you think is causing your symptoms?*" and "*What concerns or worries do you have about your condition?*"

The responses help the doctor understand the patient's inner thoughts and feelings.

6. **Elicit the patient's understanding of their symptoms and then provide a thorough explanation of the disorder that considers their views.** For example, the doctor may say, *"I understand you believe you have an infection that has not been diagnosed, but the infection is gone. However, your nerves were affected by it, so that you feel as though the infection is still there, just like a 'phantom limb.'"*
7. **Identify and respond realistically to the patient's expectations for improvement.** The doctor can say: *"How do you feel I can be helpful to you?"* This offers the opportunity for the doctor to identify expectations that can be achieved and come up with a realistic compromise. For example, if a patient has had pain for 20 years, the doctor can say that a more achievable goal might be a reduction of symptom intensity of about 30% and the ability to return to work, even with some pain.
8. **When possible, provide a link between stressors and symptoms that are consistent with the patient's understanding.** Many patients are unable or unwilling to associate stressors with illness, but most will understand that the illness causes distress and can affect their emotional state. For example, the doctor may say: *"I understand you don't see stress as causing your pain, but you've mentioned how severe and disabling your pain is. How much do you think that is causing your emotional distress?"*
9. **Set consistent limits.** Sometimes patient interests may not be compatible with optimal care. If the patient requests narcotics, the doctor can say: *"I appreciate how bad the pain must be, but narcotic medication is not helpful for chronic pain and may be harmful. Let me suggest some other options to help in the long term."*
10. **Involve the patient in the treatment.** The doctor should allow the patient to make choices. For example: *"Let me suggest some treatments for you to consider. Medication 'A' has 'B' benefits and 'C' side effects. Medication 'B' has 'D' benefits and 'E' side effects. Let's discuss the pros and cons of each so you can make a decision."*
11. **Provide explanations to help patients understand the recommendations.** For example, if the patient is reluctant to take a neuromodulator, believing it is for stress or psychiatric diagnosis, the doctor can say: *"Yes, we use antidepressants for depression, but medications can have more than one effect. Aspirin can treat pain and can also treat a heart attack. In this case, the medication can also 'turn down' the pain by blocking pain pathways through the brain-gut axis, and this benefit happens with doses lower than those used for depression."*

12. **Establish and maintain boundaries.** At times, the doctor may experience frequent phone calls, unexpected visits, tendencies to overrun visit time, or unrealistic expectations for care. These may occur because patients feel desperate or unheard, or it may reflect a need to address an ineffective communication style. Setting boundaries are done in a way that does not lead patients to feel rejected or belittled and it also must address the doctor's personal needs. For example, if a patient continues to bring up issues that overrun the visit time, the doctor can gently say: *"I see you have other important concerns, but our time has run out. To give this proper time, let's schedule another appointment in x weeks to address them properly."*

13. **Help establish an ongoing relationship with you or in association with a primary care provider.** The doctor should end the visit with: *"Whatever the result of this treatment, we can consider other options, and I will continue to work with you or your primary care provider through this."*

14. **End the visit, but not the care.** Closing the visit should only occur after the doctor asks, *"Have I answered all your questions?"* This allows the patient to reflect and bring up any final items; if the visit was properly done, there might not be any. As we've said, patients don't want to be abandoned in their care. The best way for the doctor to reinforce their commitment is to say: *"Remember that regardless of how things go, we will continue to work on this together."*

# Conclusion

WE SINCERELY HOPE that we have produced an informative book that is also enjoyable and perhaps even enlightening. We hope that we have succeeded in breaking long-held belief systems of dualistic thinking, create for you a new and very different understanding of how and why DGBI occur through dysregulation of the brain-gut axis, and then catalog them as a reference source. Also, we intended to teach the most fundamental aspects of the patient-doctor relationship: patient-centered care that requires collaboration and shared decision making. To get there, patients and providers must learn to effectively communicate with each other in ways that achieve mutual satisfaction and achievable goals in the care. We hope we have given you the tools to accomplish this. Finally, in keeping with the concept of patient-doctor collaboration, this book was written by a patient and a doctor for patients and doctors who must learn to work together to reach common goals.

We know that much more is needed to change the current healthcare paradigm. At least it is beginning in terms of new scientific knowledge. More effort is required to improve the medical curriculum by including the modern science on the DGBI, to develop programs that teach communication skills, to create collaborative patient-centered care, to incorporate this knowledge and these methods into clinical practice, and to reimburse clinicians for utilizing them adequately. Actuating these programs can re-engage patients and doctors and lead to mutual satisfaction and improved health outcomes.

The Rome Foundation (**www.theromefoundation.org**) has successfully legitimized the DGBI by establishing the diagnostic criteria, supporting innovative research, and offering high-quality books and learning tools as well as educational programs for doctors. DrossmanCare (**www.drossmancare.com**) has developed creative educational resources, including videos, workshops, and training programs, to help doctors expand their clinical skills in communication and patient-centered care. If you would like to help us with these efforts, please go to our websites or contact us for further information.

# References


1. Drossman DA, Ruddy J. Improving patient-provider relationships to improve health care. Clin Gastroenterol Hepatol 2020;18:1417–1426.
2. Drossman DA. History of Functional Gastrointestinal Symptoms and Disorders and Chronicle of the Rome Foundation. In: Drossman DA, Chang L, Chey WD, Kellow J, Tack J, Whitehead WE, eds. Rome IV Functional Gastrointestinal Disorders - Disorders of Gut-Brain Interaction. 4th ed. Raleigh, NC: Rome Foundation, 2016:549–577.
3. Drossman DA. Functional gastrointestinal disorders: History, pathophysiology, clinical features and Rome IV. Gastroenterology 2016;148:1262–1279.
4. Manning AP, Thompson WG, Heaton KW, et al. Towards positive diagnosis of the irritable bowel. Br Med J 1978;2:653–654.
5. Drossman DA. Functional Gastrointestinal Disorders and the Rome IV Process. In: Drossman DA, Chang L, Chey WD, Kellow J, Tack J, Whitehead WE, eds. Rome IV Functional Gastrointestinal Disorders - Disorders of the Gut-Brain Interaction. 4th ed. Raleigh, NC: Rome Foundation, 2016:1–32.
6. Thompson WG, Dotevall G, Drossman DA, et al. Irritable bowel syndrome: Guidelines for the diagnosis. Gastroenterology International 1989;2:92–95.
7. Drossman DA, Thompson WG, Talley NJ, et al. Identification of subgroups of functional bowel disorders. Gastroenterology International 1990;3:159–172.
8. Drossman DA. Functional GI disorders: What's in a name? Gastroenterology 2005; 128:1771–1772.
9. Kroenke K, Mangelsdorff AD. Common symptoms in ambulatory care: Incidence, evaluation, therapy, and outcome. Am J Med 1989;86:262–266.
10. Fox RC. Training for uncertainty. In: Merton R, Reader D, Kendall T, eds. The Student Physician. 1st ed. Cambridge: Harvard University Press, 1957:207–241.
11. Scarry E. The Body in Pain: The Making and Unmaking of the World. New York: Oxford University Press, 1985.
12. Engel GL. The need for a new medical model: A challenge for biomedicine. Science 1977;196:129–136.
13. Drossman DA. Presidential address: Gastrointestinal illness and biopsychosocial model. Psychosom Med 1998;60:258–267.
14. Levy RL, Whitehead WE, Von Korff MR, et al. Intergenerational transmission of gastrointestinal illness behavior. AJG 2000;95:451–456.
15. Drossman DA, Chang L, Chey WD, et al. Rome IV Functional Gastrointestinal Disorders - Disorders of Gut-Brain Interaction. 4th ed. Raleigh, NC: Rome Foundation, 2016.
16. Aziz Q, Fass R, Gyawali CP, et al. Esophageal disorders. Gastroenterology 2016; 150:1368–1379.

17. Stanghellini V, Chan FK, Hasler WL, et al. Gastroduodenal disorders. Gastroenterology 2016;150:1380–1392.
18. Lacy BE, Mearin F, Chang L, et al. Bowel disorders. Gastroenterology 2016;150: 1393–1407.
19. Keefer L, Drossman DA, Guthrie E, et al. Centrally mediated disorders of gastrointestinal pain. Gastroenterology 2016;150:1408–1419.
20. Cotton PB, Elta GH, Carter CR, et al. Gallbladder and Sphincter of Oddi disorders. Gastroenterology 2016;150:1490–1429.
21. Rao SS, Bharucha AE, Chiarioni G, et al. Functional anorectal disorders. Gastroenterology 2016;150:1430–1442.
22. Benninga MA, Faure C, Hyman PE, et al. Childhood functional gastrointestinal disorders: Neonate/toddler. Gastroenterology 2016;150:1443–1455.
23. Hyams JS, Di LC, Saps M, et al. Childhood functional gastrointestinal disorders: Children and adolescents. Gastroenterology 2016;150:1456–1468.
24. Drossman DA, Chang L, Chey WD, et al. Rome IV Functional Gastrointestinal Disorders - Disorders of Gut-Brain Interaction. 4th ed. Raleigh, NC: Rome Foundation, 2016.
25. Drossman DA, Tack J, Ford AC, et al. Neuromodulators for functional GI disorders (disorders of gut-brain interaction): A Rome Foundation Working Team Report. Gastroenterology 2018;154:1140–1171.
26. Murray HB, Juarascio AS, Di Lorenzo C, et al. Diagnosis and treatment of rumination syndrome: A critical review. Am J Gastroenterol 2019;114:562–578.
27. Keefer L, Palsson OS, Pandolfino JE. Best practice update: Incorporating psychogastroenterology into management of digestive disorders. Gastroenterology 2018;154:1249–1257.
28. Heaton KW, O'Donnell LJ. An office guide to whole-gut transit time. Patients' recollection of their stool form. J. Clin. Gastroenterol 1994;19:28–30.
29. Melzack R, Wall P. Gate-control and other mechanisms. In: Melzack R, Wall P, eds. The Challenge of Pain. 2nd ed. London: Pelican Books, 1988:165–193.
30. Ruddy J. From pretending to truly being OK: A journey from illness to health with postinfection irritable bowel syndrome: The patient's perspective. Gastroenterology 2018;155:1666–1669.
31. Drossman DA. From pretending to truly being OK: A journey from illness to health with postinfection irritable bowel syndrome: The provider's perspective. Gastroenterology 2018;155:1664–1665.
32. Drossman DA. Abuse, trauma and GI illness: Is there a link? Amer J Gastroenterol 2011;106:14–25.
33. Drossman DA, Li Z, Leserman J, Keefer FJ, Hu YJ, Toomey TC. Effects of coping on health outcome among female patients with gastrointestinal disorders. Psychosomatic Medicine 2000;62:309–317.
34. Grover M, Dorn SD, Weinland SR, et al. Atypical antipsychotic Quetiapine in the management of severe, refractory functional gastrointestinal disorders. Digestive Diseases and Sciences 2009;54:1284–1291.
35. Grunkemeier DMS, Cassara JE, Dalton CB, et al. The narcotic bowel syndrome: Clinical features, pathophysiology, and management. Clin Gastroenterol Hepatol 2007;5:1126–1139.

36. Drossman DA, Morris CB, Wrennall CE, et al. Diagnosis, characterization, and 3-month outcome after detoxification of 39 patients with narcotic bowel syndrome. American Journal of Gastroenterology 2012;107:1426–1440.
37. Heymen S, Scarlett Y, Jones K, et al. Randomized controlled trial shows biofeedback to be superior to pelvic floor exercises for fecal incontinence. Dis. Colon Rectum 2009;52:1730–1737.
38. Chiarioni G, Nardo A, Vantini I, et al. Biofeedback is superior to electrogalvanic stimulation and massage for treatment of levator ani syndrome. Gastroenterology 2010;138:1321–1329.
39. Drossman DA, Ruddy J. Communication skills in disorders of gut-brain interaction. Neurogastroenterology LATAM Reviews 2019;2:1–14.
40. Institute of Medicine. Crossing the Quality Chasm: A New Health System for the 21st Century. National Academy of Sciences, 2001.
41. Zandbelt LC, Smets EM, Oort FJ, et al. Satisfaction with the outpatient encounter: A comparison of patients' and physicians' views. J Gen Intern Med 2004;19:1088–1095.
42. Zanini C, Sarzi-Puttini P, Atzeni F, et al. Doctors' insights into the patient perspective: A qualitative study in the field of chronic pain. Biomed Res Int 2014;2014:514230.
43. Hoffmann DE, Tarzian AJ. The girl who cried pain: A bias against women in the treatment of pain. J Law Med Ethics 2001;29:13–27.
44. Merz CN. The Yentl syndrome is alive and well. Eur Heart J 2011;32:1313–1315.
45. Drossman DA, Chang L, Schneck S, et al. A focus group assessment of patient perspectives on irritable bowel syndrome and illness severity. Digestive Diseases & Sciences 2009;54:1532–1541.
46. Halpert A. Irritable bowel syndrome: Patient-provider interaction and patient education. J Clin Med 2018;7.
47. Costanzo C, Verghese A. The physical examination as ritual: Social sciences and embodiment in the context of the physical examination. Med Clin North Am 2018;102:425–431.
48. Regula CG, Miller JJ, Mauger DT, et al. Quality of care from a patient's perspective. Arch Dermatol 2007;143:1592–1593.
49. Crossing the Quality Chasm: A New Health System for the 21st Century. Washington (DC), 2001.
50. Drossman DA. 2012 David Sun lecture: Helping your patient by helping yourself: How to improve the patient-physician relationship by optimizing communication skills. American Journal of Gastroenterology 2013:521–528.
51. Drossman DA. Mind over matter in the postinfective irritable bowel. Gut 1999;44:306–307.
52. Barbara G, Grover M, Bercik P, et al. Rome Foundation Working Team Report on post-infection irritable bowel syndrome. Gastroenterology 2019;156:46–58 e7.
53. Zborowski M. Cultural components in responses to pain. J Social Issues 1952; 8:16–30.
54. Kleinman A, Eisenberg L, Good B. Culture, illness and care. Clinical lessons from anthropologic and cross-cultural research. Ann Intern Med 1978;88:251–258.
55. Toner BB, Akman D. Gender role and IBS: Literature review and hypothesis. American Journal of Gastroenterology 1999;95:11–16.

56. Ringel Y, Drossman DA, Leserman JL, et al. Effect of abuse history on pain reports and brain responses to aversive visceral stimulation: An fMRI study. Gastroenterology 2008;134:396–404.
57. Roter DL, Hall JA. Doctors talking with patients/patients talking with doctors: Improving communication in medical visits. Westport, CT: Praeger Publishing, 2006.
58. Dimatteo MR, Hays RD, Prince LM. Relationship of physicians' nonverbal communication skill to patient satisfaction, appointment noncompliance, and physician workload. Health Psychol 1986;5:581–594.
59. Wong RK, Drossman DA, Bharucha AE, et al. The digital rectal exam: A multicenter survey of physician and students' perceptions and practice patterns. American Journal of Gastroenterology 2012;107:1157–1163.
60. Kellow J, Drossman DA, et al., eds. Rome IV Diagnostic Algorithms for Common GI Symptoms. Raleigh, NC: Rome Foundation, 2016.
61. DeVaul RA, Faillace LA. Persistent pain and illness insistence: A medical profile of proneness to surgery. Am J Surg 1978;135:828–833.
62. Keefer L, Drossman DA, Guthrie E, et al. Centrally mediated disorders of gastrointestinal pain. Gastroenterology 2016;148:1408–1419.
63. Drossman DA, Chang L, Bellamy N, et al. Severity in irritable bowel syndrome: A Rome Foundation Working Team Report. Am J Gastroenterol 2011;106:1749–1759.
64. Drossman DA. Functional gastrointestinal disorders: History, pathophysiology, clinical features and Rome IV. Gastroenterology 2016;148:1262–1279.
65. Drossman DA, Chang L, Chey WD, et al. Rome IV Multidimensional Clinical Profile for Functional Gastrointestinal Disorders. Raleigh, NC: Rome Foundation, 2016.

# Glossary of Terms

**Abdominophrenic Dyssynergia**: Visible distention of the abdomen characterized by an abnormal reflex of the diaphragm and abdominal wall muscles that often, but not always, occurs after eating. It causes the diaphragm to push down and the abdominal rectus muscle to relax, which leads to the distension. This is unrelated to increased abdominal gas.

**Abuse**: Threats or actions of an emotional, sexual, or physical nature in which a power differential exists between the perpetrator and the victim

**Achalasia**: A condition in which the muscles of the lower part of the esophagus fail to relax resulting in food not passing into the stomach

**Alarm Symptoms**: Symptoms such as fever, bleeding, anemia, weight loss, or physical findings such as an abdominal mass that cannot be explained by functional gastrointestinal disorders

**Altered Mucosal and Immune Function**: Changes to the bowel's mucous membrane and immune response, e.g., "leaky gut"

**Anal Fissures**: A small tear in the thin, moist tissue that lines the anus that may occur when passing hard or large stool

**Anemia**: Low iron in the blood

**Anoscopy**: Examination of the anus and lower rectum with a rigid tube

**Antidepressant**: A class of drugs whose primary effect is to correct neurotransmitter imbalance in the central nervous system occurring in a major depression. Antidepressants tend to be useful in the DGBI to treat abdominal pain, nausea and vomiting, and concomitant anxiety and depression.

**Ascites**: An abnormal build-up of fluid in the abdomen. Most often related to liver or kidney disease or heart failure.

**Avoidance Restrictive Food Intake Disorder (ARFID)**: An eating disorder defined by severely restricting the quantity of foods eaten to the point of malnourishment

**Balloon Expulsion Test**: This is a test for dyssynergic defecation. A deflated balloon is placed in the rectum and then inflated to about 2 ounces of fluid to simulate a stool. Then while sitting privately on a commode chair, the patient is asked to expel the balloon within 2 minutes. If this does not occur the test is considered abnormal.

**Belching Disorders**: The audible escape of air from the esophagus (supragastric) or the stomach (gastric) into the pharynx. This is only considered a disorder when it is excessive and becomes troublesome.

**Biliary Pain**: Pain that is episodic and located in the upper quadrant or the epigastrium (upper central region) of the abdomen that lasts 30 minutes or longer and is severe enough to interrupt daily activities or lead to an emergency room visit

**Biofeedback Treatment**: The use of electronic or mechanical devices to provide visual and/or auditory information (feedback) on a biological process for the purpose of teaching an individual to control the biological process. Generalized biofeedback provides information about large muscles of the body to achieve generalized relaxation. Anorectal biofeedback allows relaxation of the rectal muscles. Pressure sensors or EMG are placed inside the anus and rectum to provide feedback to the patient on muscle activity during simulated defecation.

**Biomedical Model**: The model of illness and disease in Western medical education and research. It has two assumptions: (1) mind and body are separate (dualism), and (2) illness and disease originate from a single cause (biomedical reductionism)

**Biomedical Reductionism**: The concept that all disease can be reduced to a single etiology or biological cause

**Biopsychosocial**: The concept that illness and disease result from the combined influence of biological, psychosocial, and social factors. The brain and the body interact.

**Biopsychosocial Model**: A model that proposes that illness and disease result from simultaneously interacting systems at the cellular, tissue, organismal, interpersonal, and environmental level. It incorporates the biological aspects of the disorder with the unique psychosocial features of the individual, and it helps explain the variability in symptom expression among individuals having the same biological condition.

**Bloating**: A sensation of discomfort or fullness in the abdomen. It may or may not be accompanied by visible abdominal distension.

**Calprotectin Test**: A stool test used to detect inflammation in the intestines. This is a test to screen for inflammatory bowel disease.

**Cannabinoid Hyperemesis Syndrome (CHS)**: Episodes of vomiting similar to cyclic vomiting syndrome (CVS) in their onset, duration, and frequency. These episodes occur after prolonged, excessive cannabis use and stop when cannabis use is discontinued.

**Catastrophizing**: A type of unhelpful thinking. Catastrophic thoughts tend to dwell on the worst possible outcome of any situation in which there is a possibility of an unpleasant outcome (e.g., a person taking an airplane dwells on the possibility of the airplane crashing).

**CBC**: Complete blood count. This tests for anemia (red cells), inflammation (white cells), and clotting tendency (platelets).

**Celiac Disease**: A disease that may present similar to IBS but is due to an allergy to gluten, a protein found in wheat, barley, and rye. It is treated by reducing gluten in the diet.

**Centrally Mediated Abdominal Pain Syndrome (CAPS)**: Continuous, nearly continuous, or frequently recurrent abdominal pain that is often severe and not or rarely related to changes in gut function such as eating or defecation. The pain is not feigned or related to another gastrointestinal disorder. The chronic and severe pain associated is a hallmark complaint.

**Chronic Nausea Vomiting Syndrome**: Nausea occurring at least 1 day a week that is severe enough to impact usual activities, and one or more vomiting episodes a week. However, nausea can occur without vomiting. Eating disorders and self-induced vomiting must be excluded, and tests (including an upper endoscopy) find no evidence of organic abnormality.

**Coccygodynia**: Pain in or around the bony structure called the coccyx at the base of the spine

**Cognitive Behavioral Therapy (CBT)**: Several approaches or sets of techniques used by mental health professionals. CBT focuses on challenging and changing unhelpful cognitive distortions (e.g., thoughts, beliefs, and attitudes) and behaviors, improving emotional regulation, and the development of personal coping strategies that target solving current problems. It has been proven successful in treating DGBI.

**Colonoscopy**: An endoscopic examination of the lining of the colon to find polyps or inflammation

**Colon Polyp**: An abnormal growth in the lining of the colon that can develop into a cancer. This more often occurs when there is a tubular adenoma ≥10 mm in size, an adenoma of any size with villous features or high-grade dysplasia, or a dysplastic serrated lesion of any size.

**Co-Morbidity**: The simultaneous presence of two chronic diseases or conditions in a patient

**C-Reactive Protein Blood Test**: A blood test that checks for inflammation in the body

**Crohn's Disease**: A chronic inflammatory bowel disease characterized by inflammation or ulceration of the colon or small intestine that can be complicated by bleeding, obstruction, or infection. This needs to be excluded in patients presenting with functional bowel complaints of pain and diarrhea.

**Cyclic Vomiting Syndrome (CVS)**: A functional gastroduodenal disorder characterized by intermittent stereotypical episodes of intense nausea and vomiting (up to 30 times a day) that may occur multiple times a year, lasting for a week or more, and the absence of nausea and vomiting between episodes

**Defecography**: An x-ray or MRI technique that provides a detailed view of the anatomy and functioning of the rectum and pelvic floor before and during attempted defecation

**Disorder of Gut-Brain Interaction (DGBI)**: This was formerly called a Functional GI Disorder. DGBI more appropriately identifies these disorders as dysregulation of the brain-gut axis. Patients with these disorders may have visceral hypersensitivity, altered mucosal immune function, altered microbiota, or central dysregulation.

**Diverticulitis**: The infection or inflammation of the pouches that can form in the colon

**Dysphagia**: Difficulty swallowing without pain

**Dyssynergic Defecation**: A functional anorectal disorder caused by inappropriate or paradoxical contraction of the pelvic floor with failure to relax the levator muscle (puborectalis), associated with straining and difficulty evacuating

**Ejection Fraction**: Ejection fraction (EF) is a measurement, expressed as a percentage, of how much the gallbladder empties after contracting. An ejection fraction of less than 40% is suggestive of functional gallbladder disorder

**Empiric Value**: Based on practical experience instead of scientific proof

**Enterocele**: Descent of loops of small intestine into the pelvis that bulge into the vagina during straining. An enterocele may cause pain, a sensation of fullness, and/or obstructed defecation.

**Eosinophilic Esophagitis (EOE)**: A chronic, inflammatory disease of the esophagus associated with large numbers of eosinophils. This disorder may be dietary or allergic related.

**Eosinophils**: A type of inflammatory cell that can be seen in increased numbers in allergies or parasitic infections. It is increased in eosinophilic esophagitis and in certain types of functional dyspepsia.

**Epigastric Pain Syndrome (EPS)**: A subtype of functional dyspepsia characterized by epigastric pain or burning that may or may not occur in relation to meals

**Esophagogastric Junction (EGJ):** The esophagogastric junction is the region between the distal esophagus and the upper part or cardia of the stomach. The lower esophageal sphincter is located. Contraction of this sphincter prevents the esophagus from getting acid. A weak sphincter with GERD leads to esophagitis and inflammation.

**Esophageal Spasm**: Increased contractions of the esophagus that can be seen by barium swallow x-ray or by esophageal manometry

**Etiology**: The cause, set of causes, or manner of causation of a disease or condition

**Excessive Supragastric Belching (From Esophagus)**: Excessive belching that occurs more than 3 days a week, caused by gas that originates from air swallowing into the esophagus, which is then released

**Excessive Gastric Belching (From Stomach)**: Excessive belching that occurs more than 3 days a week, caused by air swallowing into the stomach, which is then released

**Fecal Elastase**: A stool test to determine if there is pancreatic insufficiency causing diarrhea. The pancreas produces elastase so the elastase value is decreased in pancreatic insufficiency.

**Fecal Incontinence**: Recurrent uncontrolled passage of fecal material for at least 3 months

**Feigned**: Consciously faked

**Fibromyalgia**: A chronic disorder characterized by widespread musculoskeletal pain, fatigue, and tenderness in localized areas

**Functional Abdominal Bloating/Distension**: A functional bowel disorder characterized by recurrent bloating and distension of the abdomen that occurs on average at least 1 day a week and predominates over other symptoms. To make this diagnosis by Rome Criteria, other DGBI should be excluded.

**Functional Anorectal Pain**: A functional anorectal disorder characterized by pain in the anorectal area, which is primarily distinguished by the duration of pain and the presence or absence of anorectal tenderness

**Functional Biliary Sphincter of Oddi (SO) Disorder**: A functional biliary disorder characterized by biliary pain in the absence of bile duct stones or other structural abnormalities that is associated with abnormal liver enzymes or a dilated bile duct (but not both). Often, the gallbladder has been surgically removed.

**Functional Chest Pain**: A functional esophageal disorder characterized by recurring, unexplained chest pain behind the sternum that is not experienced as heartburn but is believed to be related to the esophagus. Heart disease should be excluded by medical evaluation or cardiac diagnostic studies.

**Functional Constipation**: A functional bowel disorder characterized by difficult defecation and infrequent or incomplete bowel movements. Abdominal pain or bloating may be present but do not predominate (as they do with IBS-C).

**Functional Defecation Disorders (FDD)**: A functional anorectal disorder that is also called pelvic floor dyssynergia. It is characterized by frequent excessive straining, feeling of incomplete evacuation with defecation, and at times digital facilitation of bowel movements. The pelvic floor muscles contract with defecation, rather than relaxing, as they should, or there is not enough pressure (propulsive force) to defecate.

**Functional Diarrhea**: A functional bowel disorder characterized by loose or watery stools, without predominant abdominal pain or bothersome bloating, occurring 25% of the time or more. Patients meeting criteria for IBS-D should be excluded.

**Functional Dyspepsia**: A functional gastroduodenal disorder in which any of the following apply: the unpleasant sensation of food staying in the stomach after a meal ("postprandial fullness"); the unpleasant feeling that the stomach is overfilled soon after starting to eat ("early satiety"); subjective, intense pain in the area just above the stomach ("epigastric pain"); and/or unpleasant, subjective sensation of heat in the epigastrium. These symptoms significantly impact usual activities.

**Functional Dysphagia**: A functional gastroduodenal disorder characterized by a sense of solid and/or liquid foods sticking, lodging, or passing abnormally through the esophagus

**Functional Gallbladder Disorder**: A functional gallbladder disorder characterized by biliary pain in the absence of gallstones or other structural pathology. It may be diagnosed by a low ejection fraction.

**Functional Heartburn**: A functional esophageal disorder characterized by burning discomfort or pain (i.e., heartburn) experienced behind the breastbone (retro-sternal) that is not associated with increased acid reflux. It does not respond to acid-blocking treatments and is not caused by any structural diagnosis like GERD or a motility disorder.

**Functional Pancreatic SO Disorder**: A functional Sphincter of Oddi disorder characterized by biliary pain associated with increased pressures in the pancreatic duct leading to inflammation of the pancreas and elevated pancreatic enzymes. These patients may be treated by endoscopic sphincterotomy.

**Gastric Inlet Patch**: A congenital anomaly consisting of gastric mucosa at or just distal to the upper esophageal sphincter

**Gastroduodenal Disorders**: A class of DGBI involving symptoms that are attributed to the stomach and the duodenum (the first part of the small intestine, immediately beneath the stomach)

**Globus**: A functional esophageal disorder characterized by the persistent or intermittent non-painful sensation of a lump or foreign body in the throat. It occurs episodically and is felt in the midline above the sternal notch.

**Gut Microbiota**: The microorganisms found in the intestines or gut

***H. pylori* Infection**: A type of bacteria that produces inflammation and ulcers in the stomach. This may produce symptoms consistent with functional dyspepsia and if found may be eradicated with antibiotics.

**Hematochezia**: The passage of bright red blood via the anus

**Ileus**: The loss of normal peristalsis or contractions of the bowel, which can be due to motility disorders such as pseudo-obstruction, after abdominal surgery, or after certain types of medications that slow down motility

**Inadequate Defecatory Propulsion**: A type of anorectal disorder characterized by inadequate propulsive force of the rectum preventing proper defecation

**Intraluminal Impedance**: A type of test usually done with pH (acid) testing to evaluate heartburn. It is based on the measurement of changes in resistance to alternating electrical current when a bolus passes by a pair of metallic rings mounted on a catheter.

**Irritable Bowel Syndrome (IBS)**: A functional bowel disorder characterized by recurrent abdominal pain that is related to defecation and associated with constipation, diarrhea, or a mixture of both; abdominal bloating and distension may also be present. The IBS subtypes C, D, M, and U are differentiated by relative frequencies of the stool form.

**Levator Ani Syndrome**: A type of anorectal disorder characterized by rectal pain that is often described as a vague, dull ache, or a sensation of pressure high in the rectum lasting 30 minutes or longer. It is often worse when sitting than when standing or lying down. Physical examination reveals tenderness when the doctor presses on the pelvic floor (posterior traction of the levator) muscle. Other structural disorders of the pelvic floor must be excluded.

**Lipase Test**: A blood test that measures a type of protein (lipase) in the blood that is produced by the pancreas. It is a way to diagnose pancreatitis based on elevated blood levels.

**Manometry**: Anorectal manometric (ARM) measures the anal and rectal pressures and EMG (electromyogram) electrical activity during attempted defecation. When these tests are normal, increased intrarectal pressure is associated with anal relaxation. An abnormal study will demonstrate inappropriately increased pressures or inadequate relaxation of the rectum or the anal sphincter during simulated defecation.

**Microbiota**: All the microorganisms (bacteria, yeast, fungi, viruses) living in a specific environment, called a microbiome

**Mind-Body Dualism**: A concept promoted by René Descartes in the 17th century that promotes the separation of the mind and the body. In Western medicine this has led to a distinction between "organic," i.e., structural disorders or "functional," i.e., not structural disorders that are considered less legitimate. It has promoted the misunderstanding of DGBI as psychiatric or not real and is challenged by the biopsychosocial model.

**Motility Disturbance or Dysmotility**: Disorders that are characterized by abnormal movement inside the bowels

**Narcotic Bowel Syndrome (NBS) / Opioid-Induced GI Hyperalgesia**: A centrally mediated disorder of GI pain characterized by the development of (or increases in) abdominal pain associated with continuous or increasing dosages of opioids. The pain is not explained by other medical diagnoses. When opioid use ends, improvement or resolution will occur.

**Nausea**: Queasiness or sick sensation. It is the unpleasant sensation of needing to vomit, typically felt in the upper abdomen immediately above the stomach or throat.

**Nausea and Vomiting Disorder**: Chronic nausea and vomiting disorder (CNVS) is a functional gastroduodenal disorder related to chronic nausea, vomiting, or both

**Neuroplastic**: A characteristic of the plasticity of nerve cells indicating that they can grow (neurogenesis) and shrink (neurodegeneration)

**Odynophagia**: Painful swallowing

**Opioid-Induced Constipation**: New or worsening symptoms of constipation when initiating, changing, or increasing opioid therapy

**Orthorexia**: The disordered thought process that certain foods are producing unwanted symptoms or health impairments that lead to food restriction

**Pancreaticobiliary Disease**: Disorders of the gall bladder, biliary ducts, and pancreas

**Pathophysiology**: The physiological understanding of how and why medical disorders are occurring

**Patient-Doctor Relationship**: Ideally understood in terms of interpersonal behaviors that enhance or diminish mutual communication, satisfaction, and trust. Positive physician behaviors are characterized by empathy, respect, and positive regard.

**Pelvic Floor**: The pelvic floor relates to the rectal and urogenital region of the human body. It is composed of muscle fibers of the levator ani, the coccygeus muscle, and associated connective tissues that span the area underneath the pelvis. The pelvic floor separates the pelvic cavity above from the perineal region (including perineum) below. Because, to accommodate the birth canal, a female's pelvic cavity is larger than a male's, the pelvic floor tends to be considered a part of female anatomy, but males have an equivalent pelvic floor.

**Peristalsis**: The involuntary constriction and relaxation of the muscles of the intestine or another canal, creating wave-like movements that push the contents forward through the GI tract

**Polyposis Syndrome**: A hereditary condition that is associated with an increased risk of developing polyps in the digestive tract, most commonly in the colon and/or rectum. A polyp is a growth of normal tissue that forms a lump. As the name suggests, a variety of polyps may occur.

**Postprandial Distress Syndrome (PDS)**: A subtype of functional dyspepsia. It is characterized by the uncomfortable sensation of being too full soon after eating a meal or becoming full so early that eating a regular-sized meal is prevented. PDS is characterized exclusively by meal-induced symptoms.

**Postural Orthostatic Tachycardia Syndrome (POTS)**: This is a functional vascular disorder commonly associated with some DGBI. It relates to an abnormal increase in heart rate or blood pressure that occurs after sitting up or standing. Some typical symptoms include dizziness and fainting. It is related to abnormal regulation of the autonomic nervous system.

**Proctalgia Fugax**: This is a functional anorectal disorder characterized by recurrent episodes of pain in the rectal area, lasting for a few seconds to several minutes (up to 30 minutes) and then disappearing completely. The pain is usually localized to the rectum; it has been described as cramping, gnawing, aching, or stabbing; and may range from uncomfortable to unbearable.

**Proton Pump Inhibitors (PPI)**: Medications designed to decrease acid secretions. Examples include Prilosec (omeprazole), Nexium (esomeprazole), and Protonix (pantoprazole).

**Pseudo-Obstruction**: Intestinal pseudo-obstruction is caused by nerve or muscle problems that prevent the intestines from contracting normally to move food, fluid, and air through the intestines. Symptoms may include cramps, abdominal pain, nausea, vomiting, bloating, constipation, and occasionally diarrhea.

**Rectal Prolapse**: Protrusion of the mucosal lining of the rectum through the anus

**Rectoanal Reflex**: The rectoanal inhibitory reflex (RAIR) is a reflex characterized by a transient involuntary relaxation of the internal anal sphincter in response to distention of the rectum. When difficulties occur with proper relaxation, we call this dyssynergic defecation.

**Rectocele**: A weakening of the wall between the rectum and vagina. It can develop from weakness in the wall from multiple vaginal deliveries or surgeries or repeated straining leading to increased abdominal pressure generated that pushes the rectal wall into the vaginal area.

**Reflux Hypersensitivity**: Heartburn or chest pain when endoscopy and pH studies are normal, but symptoms occur when acid enters the esophagus. This is not GERD because esophageal pH testing shows no increased acid, but the esophagus is found to be sensitive to acid.

**Retrosternal**: Located behind the breastbone, or sternum

**Rome Criteria**: Lists of symptoms in which a specified minimum number allows a diagnosis of a DGBI. The criteria change over time depending on scientific investigation. Rome IV are the current criteria.

**Rumination Syndrome**: A functional gastroduodenal disorder characterized by repetitive, effortless regurgitation of recently eaten food into the mouth, which is then re-swallowed or spit out. Regurgitation is not preceded by retching and occurs before the food has turned into acid.

**Sacral Nerve Stimulation**: An implant that delivers gentle electrical impulses through a probe (a thin wire) that is placed near the sacral nerve. The technology is similar to a pacemaker, but instead of regulating a person's heartbeat, it stimulates the bowel, sphincter, and bladder muscles to work normally. It is used to treat fecal incontinence.

**Satiation**: The feeling after eating of being full

**Scintigraph**: Also known as a gamma scan, this is a diagnostic test in nuclear medicine where radioisotopes attached to drugs that travel to a specific organ or tissue (radiopharmaceuticals) are taken internally, and the emitted gamma radiation is captured by external detectors (gamma cameras) to form two-dimensional images in a similar process to the capture of x-ray images

**Scintigraphic Test**: A test to evaluate slow gallbladder emptying (CCK-CS) involving the intravenous administration of technetium 99m (Tc 99m), which is excreted into the biliary tract and concentrated in the GB. The rate to which the Tc 99m empties out of the gallbladder is called the ejection fraction (EF). If the EF is low (usually 40% or less), the diagnosis is supported.

**Secretagogues**: A class of drugs to treat constipation and IBS-C that increase fluid into the intestines to produce a more frequent, softer stool, and to reduce bloating

**Sitaphobia**: Fear of eating due to unwanted side effects, usually pain

**Sitzmarker/Intramarx Test**: A sitz marker study is where capsules containing small radio opaque markers are ingested to evaluate how quickly they move through the colon. The capsules may done at one time, and daily after 3 or 5 days, and then an abdominal x-ray is taken. This test is most often used with patients who are suffering from chronic constipation.

**Splinting**: A technique where the patient uses a finger to push up and back either at the back of the vagina or in the area between the vagina and rectum. This straightens the anorectal angle to allow for easier passage of stool. Splinting is commonly used as a treatment for patients who have a rectocele.

**Stricture**: An abnormal narrowing of a bodily passage (as from inflammation, cancer, or the formation of scar tissue)

**Unspecified Functional Anorectal Pain**: A type of anorectal disorder characterized by the same symptoms as Levator Ani Syndrome, but upon rectal exam there is no tenderness when the doctor presses on the levator muscle

**Unspecified Functional Bowel Disorder**: A type of functional bowel disorder where bowel symptoms, including abdominal pain or change in bowel habits, do not have an organic cause and do not meet criteria for IBS or functional constipation, diarrhea, or abdominal bloating/distention disorders

**Upper Endocosopy**: A test in which a thin scope with a camera is used to look inside the esophagus, stomach, and duodenum

**Vagal Nerve**: This is the 10th cranial nerve that carries information between the brain and other organs of the body including the GI tract, heart, and lung. It is a parasympathetic nerve bringing information from and to the digestive organs.

**Vasovagal Reflex**: An abnormal reflex that can occur causing problems like a drop in blood pressure or abdominophrenic dyssynergia; it may relate to increased autonomic reactivity

**Visceral Hypersensitivity**: One of the main features of IBS and some other DGBI where there is increased firing of nerves in the digestive tract after stimulation or stretching of the bowel. This produces a lower pain threshold and explains why patients with DGBI may get pain after eating.

**Vomiting**: Vomiting is the forceful oral expulsion of gastrointestinal contents associated with contraction of the abdominal and chest wall muscles; it is usually associated with nausea

APPENDIX A

# Rome IV Diagnostic Criteria

## A. Esophageal Disorders

### A1. Functional Chest Pain

*Diagnostic criteria* Must include **all** of the following:*

1. Retrosternal chest pain or discomfort**
2. Absence of associated esophageal symptoms, such as heartburn and dysphagia
3. Absence of evidence that gastroesophageal reflux or eosinophilic esophagitis is the cause of the symptom
4. Absence of major esophageal motor disorders†

* Criteria fulfilled for the last 3 months with symptom onset at least 6 months prior to diagnosis with a frequency of at least once a week

** Cardiac causes should be ruled out

† Achalasia/EGJ outflow obstruction, diffuse esophageal spasm, jackhammer esophagus, absent peristalsis

### A2. Functional Heartburn

*Diagnostic criteria* Must include **all** of the following:*

1. Burning retrosternal discomfort or pain
2. No symptom relief despite optimal antisecretory therapy
3. Absence of evidence that gastroesophageal reflux** or eosinophilic esophagitis is the cause of the symptom
4. Absence of major esophageal motor disorders†

* Criteria fulfilled for the last 3 months with symptom onset at least 6 months prior to diagnosis with a frequency of at least twice a week

** Elevated acid exposure time and/or symptom reflux association

† Achalasia/EGJ outflow obstruction, diffuse esophageal spasm, jackhammer esophagus, absent peristalsis

### A3. Reflux Hypersensitivity

*Diagnostic criteria* Must include **all** of the following:*

1. Retrosternal symptoms including heartburn and chest pain
2. Normal endoscopy and absence of evidence that eosinophilic esophagitis is the cause of the symptoms
3. Absence of major esophageal motor disorders**
4. Evidence of triggering of symptoms by reflux events despite normal acid exposure on pH or pH-impedance monitoring†

* Criteria fulfilled for the last 3 months with symptom onset at least 6 months prior to diagnosis with a frequency of at least twice a week

** Achalasia/EGJ outflow obstruction, diffuse esophageal spasm, jackhammer esophagus, absent peristalsis

† Response to antisecretory therapy does not exclude the diagnosis

### A4. Globus

*Diagnostic criteria* Must include **all** of the following:*

1. Persistent or intermittent, non-painful sensation of a lump or foreign body in the throat with no structural lesion identified on physical examination, laryngoscopy, or endoscopy
   a. Occurrence of the sensation between meals
   b. Absence of dysphagia or odynophagia
   c. Absence of a gastric inlet patch in the proximal esophagus
2. Absence of evidence that gastroesophageal reflux or eosinophilic esophagitis is the cause of the symptom
3. Absence of major esophageal motor disorders**

* Criteria fulfilled for the last 3 months with symptom onset at least 6 months prior to diagnosis with a frequency of at least once a week

** Achalasia/EGJ outflow obstruction, diffuse esophageal spasm, jackhammer esophagus, absent peristalsis

### A5. Functional Dysphagia

*Diagnostic criteria* Must include **all** of the following:*

1. Sense of solid and/or liquid foods sticking, lodging, or passing abnormally through the esophagus
2. Absence of evidence that esophageal mucosal or structural abnormality is the cause of the symptom
3. Absence of evidence that gastroesophageal reflux or eosinophilic esophagitis is the cause of the symptom
4. Absence of major esophageal motor disorders**

* Criteria fulfilled for the last 3 months with symptom onset at least 6 months prior to diagnosis with a frequency of at least once a week

** Achalasia/EGJ outflow obstruction, diffuse esophageal spasm, jackhammer esophagus, absent peristalsis

## B. Gastroduodenal Disorders

### B1. FUNCTIONAL DYSPEPSIA* (FD)

*Diagnostic criteria***

1. ***One or more*** of the following:
   a. Bothersome postprandial fullness
   b. Bothersome early satiation
   c. Bothersome epigastric pain
   d. Bothersome epigastric burning

AND

2. No evidence of structural disease (including at upper endoscopy) that is likely to explain the symptoms

* Must fulfill criteria for B1a. PDS and/or B1b. EPS

** Criteria fulfilled for the last 3 months with symptom onset at least 6 months prior to diagnosis

## B1a. Postprandial Distress Syndrome (PDS)

*Diagnostic criteria** *Must include* ***one or both*** *of the following at least 3 days a week:*

1. Bothersome postprandial fullness (i.e., severe enough to impact on usual activities)
2. Bothersome early satiation (i.e., severe enough to prevent finishing a regular size meal)

No evidence of organic, systemic, or metabolic disease that is likely to explain the symptoms on routine investigations (including at upper endoscopy)

* Criteria fulfilled for the last 3 months with symptom onset at least 6 months prior to diagnosis

*Supportive criteria*

1. Postprandial epigastric pain or burning, epigastric bloating, excessive belching, and nausea can also be present
2. Vomiting warrants consideration of another disorder
3. Heartburn is not a dyspeptic symptom but may often co-exist
4. Symptoms that are relieved by evacuation of feces or gas should generally not be considered as part of dyspepsia
5. Other individual digestive symptoms or groups of symptoms (e.g., from GERD and IBS) may co-exist with PDS

## B1b. Epigastric Pain Syndrome (EPS)

*Diagnostic criteria** *Must include* ***one or both*** *of the following symptoms at least 1 day a week:*

1. Bothersome epigastric pain (i.e., severe enough to impact on usual activities)
2. Bothersome epigastric burning (i.e., severe enough to impact on usual activities)

No evidence of organic, systemic, or metabolic disease that is likely to explain the symptoms on routine investigations (including at upper endoscopy)

* Criteria fulfilled for the last 3 months with symptom onset at least 6 months prior to diagnosis

*Supportive criteria*

1. Pain may be induced by ingestion of a meal, relieved by ingestion of a meal, or may occur while fasting
2. Postprandial epigastric bloating, belching, and nausea can also be present
3. Persistent vomiting likely suggests another disorder
4. Heartburn is not a dyspeptic symptom but may often co-exist
5. The pain does not fulfill biliary pain criteria
6. Symptoms that are relieved by evacuation of feces or gas generally should not be considered as part of dyspepsia
7. Other digestive symptoms (such as from GERD and IBS) may co-exist with EPS

## B2. BELCHING DISORDERS

*Diagnostic criteria**

Bothersome (i.e., severe enough to impact on usual activities) belching from the esophagus or stomach more than 3 days a week

### B2a. Excessive Supragastric Belching (from esophagus)

### B2b. Excessive Gastric Belching (from stomach)

*Supportive criteria*

1. Supragastric belching is supported by observing frequent, repetitive belching
2. Gastric belching has no established clinical correlate
3. Objective intraluminal impedance measurement is required to distinguish supragastric from gastric belching

* Criteria fulfilled for the last 3 months with symptom onset at least 6 months prior to diagnosis

## B3. NAUSEA AND VOMITING DISORDERS

### B3a. Chronic Nausea Vomiting Syndrome

*Diagnostic criteria** *Must include **all** of the following:*

1. Bothersome (i.e., severe enough to impact on usual activities) nausea, occurring at least 1 day per week and/or one or more vomiting episodes per week
2. Self-induced vomiting, eating disorders, regurgitation, or rumination are excluded
3. No evidence of organic, systemic, or metabolic diseases likely to explain the symptoms on routine investigations (including at upper endoscopy)

* Criteria fulfilled for the last 3 months with symptom onset at least 6 months prior to diagnosis

### B3b. Cyclic Vomiting Syndrome (CVS)

*Diagnostic criteria** *Must include **all** of the following:*

1. Stereotypical episodes of vomiting regarding onset (*acute*) and duration (*less than 1 week*)
2. At least three discrete episodes in the prior year and two episodes in the past 6 months, occurring at least 1 week apart
3. Absence of vomiting between episodes, but other milder symptoms can be present between cycles

* Criteria fulfilled for the last 3 months with symptom onset at least 6 months prior to diagnosis

*Supportive remark*

History or family history of migraine headaches

### B3c. Cannabinoid Hyperemesis Syndrome

*Diagnostic criteria** *Must include **all** of the following:*

1. Stereotypical episodic vomiting resembling cyclic vomiting syndrome (CVS) in terms of onset, duration, and frequency
2. Presentation after prolonged use of cannabis
3. Relief of vomiting episodes by sustained cessation of cannabis use

* Criteria fulfilled for the last 3 months with symptom onset at least 6 months prior to diagnosis

*Supportive remark*

May be associated with pathologic bathing behavior (*prolonged hot baths or showers*)

### B4. Rumination Syndrome

*Diagnostic criteria** *Must include **all** of the following:*

1. Persistent or recurrent regurgitation of recently ingested food into the mouth with subsequent spitting or remastication and swallowing
2. Regurgitation is not preceded by retching

* Criteria fulfilled for the last 3 months with symptom onset at least 6 months prior to diagnosis

*Supportive criteria*

1. Effortless regurgitation events are usually not preceded by nausea
2. Regurgitant contains recognizable food which may have a pleasant taste
3. The process tends to cease when the regurgitated material becomes acidic

## C. Bowel Disorders

### C1. Irritable Bowel Syndrome (IBS)

*Diagnostic criteria**

Recurrent abdominal pain on average at least 1 day/week in the last 3 months, associated with ***two or more*** of the following criteria:

1. Related to defecation
2. Associated with a change in frequency of stool
3. Associated with a change in form (appearance) of stool

* Criteria fulfilled for the last 3 months with symptom onset at least 6 months prior to diagnosis

**IBS Subtypes** (next page)

### Diagnostic Criteria for IBS Subtypes

Predominant bowel habits are based on stool form on days with at least one abnormal bowel movement.*

**IBS with predominant constipation (IBS-C):** > ¼ (25%) of bowel movements with Bristol stool types 1 or 2 and < ¼ (25%) of bowel movements with Bristol stool types 6 or 7. *Alternative for epidemiology or clinical practice: Patient reports that abnormal bowel movements are usually constipation (like Type 1 or 2 in the picture of BSF, see figure below).*

**IBS with predominant diarrhea (IBS-D):** > ¼ (25%) of bowel movements with Bristol stool types 6 or 7 and < ¼ (25%) of bowel movements with Bristol stool types 1 or 2. *Alternative for epidemiology or clinical practice: Patient reports that abnormal bowel movements are usually diarrhea (like Type 6 or 7 in the picture of BSF, see second figure below).*

**IBS with mixed bowel habits (IBS-M):** > ¼ (25%) of bowel movements with Bristol stool types 1 or 2 and > ¼ (25%) of bowel movements with Bristol stool types 6 or 7. *Alternative for epidemiology or clinical practice: Patient reports that abnormal bowel movements are usually both constipation and diarrhea (more than ¼ of all the abnormal bowel movements were constipation and more than ¼ were diarrhea, using picture of BSF, see figure below).*

**IBS Unclassified (IBS-U):** Patients who meet diagnostic criteria for IBS but whose bowel habits cannot be accurately categorized into 1 of the 3 groups above should be categorized as having IBS-U. *Alternative for epidemiology or clinical practice: Patient reports that abnormal stools (both diarrhea and constipation) are rare.*

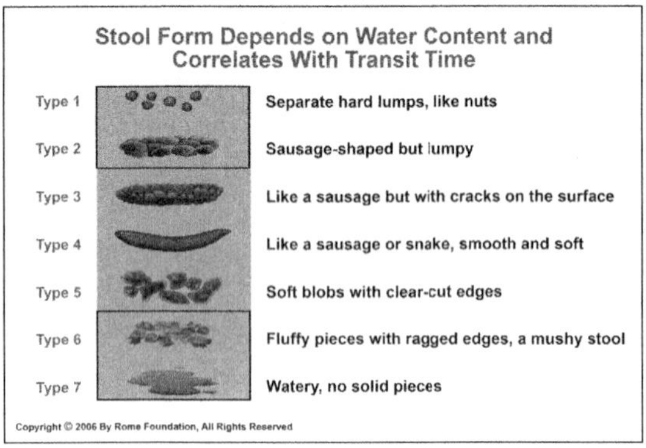



For clinical trials, subtyping based on at least 2 weeks of daily diary data is recommended, using the "25%-rule."

* IBS subtypes related to bowel habit abnormalities (IBS-C, IBS-D, and IBS-M) can only be confidently established when the patient is evaluated off medications used to treat bowel habit abnormalities.

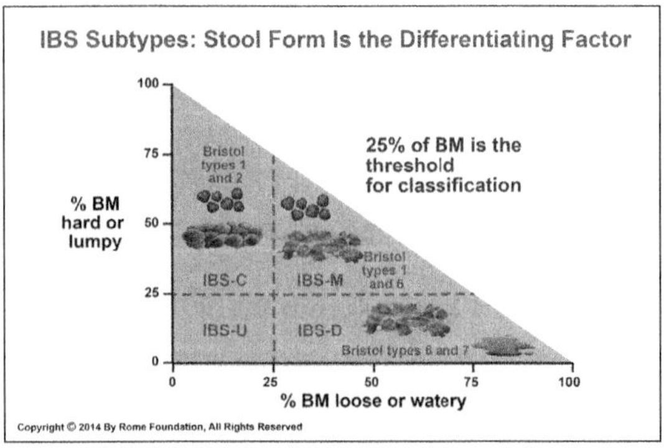

### C2. Functional Constipation (FC)

*Diagnostic criteria**

1. Must include ***two or more*** of the following:**
   a. Straining during more than ¼ (25%) of defecations
   b. Lumpy or hard stools (Bristol Stool Form Scale 1-2) more than ¼ (25%) of defecations
   c. Sensation of incomplete evacuation more than ¼ (25%) of defecations
   d. Sensation of anorectal obstruction/blockage more than ¼ (25%) of defecations
   e. Manual maneuvers to facilitate more than ¼ (25%) of defecations (e.g., digital evacuation, support of the pelvic floor)
   f. Fewer than three SBM per week
2. Loose stools are rarely present without the use of laxatives
3. Insufficient criteria for irritable bowel syndrome

* Criteria fulfilled for the last 3 months with symptom onset at least 6 months prior to diagnosis

** For research studies, patients meeting criteria for opioid-induced constipation (OIC) should not be given a diagnosis of FC because it is difficult to distinguish between opioid side effects and other causes of constipation. However, clinicians recognize that these two conditions may overlap.

### C3. Functional Diarrhea

*Diagnostic criterion**

Loose or watery stools, without predominant abdominal pain or bothersome bloating, occurring in more than 25% of stools**

* Criterion fulfilled for the last 3 months with symptom onset at least 6 months prior to diagnosis

** Patients meeting criteria for IBS-D (diarrhea-predominant IBS) should be excluded

### C4. Functional Abdominal Bloating/Distension

*Diagnostic criteria**   *Must include **both** of the following:*

1. Recurrent bloating and/or distension occurring on average at least 1 day/week; abdominal bloating and/or distension predominates over other symptoms**
2. There are insufficient criteria for a diagnosis of irritable bowel syndrome, functional constipation, functional diarrhea, or postprandial distress syndrome

* Criteria fulfilled for the last 3 months with symptom onset at least 6 months prior to diagnosis

** Mild pain related to bloating may be present as well as minor bowel movement abnormalities

### C5. Unspecified Functional Bowel Disorder

*Diagnostic criterion**

Bowel symptoms not attributable to an organic etiology that do not meet criteria for IBS, or functional constipation, diarrhea, or abdominal bloating/distension disorders

* Criterion fulfilled for the last 3 months with symptom onset at least 6 months prior to diagnosis

### C6. Opioid-Induced Constipation (OIC)

*Diagnostic criteria*

1. New, or worsening, symptoms of constipation when initiating, changing, or increasing opioid therapy, that must include ***two or more*** of the following:
   a. Straining during more than ¼ (25%) of defecations
   b. Lumpy or hard stools (Bristol Stool Form Scale 1-2) more than ¼ (25%) of defecations
   c. Sensation of incomplete evacuation more than ¼ (25%) of defecations
   d. Sensation of anorectal obstruction/blockage more than ¼ (25%) of defecations
   e. Manual maneuvers to facilitate more than ¼ (25%) of defecations (e.g., digital evacuation, support of the pelvic floor)
   f. Fewer than three SBM per week
2. Loose stools are rarely present without the use of laxatives

## D. Centrally Mediated Disorders of GI Pain

### D1. Centrally Mediated Abdominal Pain Syndrome* (CAPS)

*Diagnostic criteria*** *Must include* ***all*** *of the following:*

1. Continuous or nearly continuous abdominal pain
2. No or only occasional relationship of pain with physiological events (e.g., eating, defecation, or menses)†
3. Pain limits some aspect of daily functioning††
4. The pain is not feigned
5. Pain is not explained by another structural or functional gastrointestinal disorder or other medical condition

* CAPS is typically associated with psychosocial comorbidity, but there is no specific profile that can be used for diagnosis

** Criteria fulfilled for the last 3 months with symptom onset at least 6 months prior to diagnosis

† Some degree of gastrointestinal dysfunction may be present

†† Daily function could include impairments in work, intimacy, social/leisure, family life, and caregiving for self or others

### D2. Narcotic Bowel Syndrome/Opioid-Induced GI Hyperalgesia

*Diagnostic criteria* *Must include **all** of the following:*

1. Chronic or frequently recurring abdominal pain* that is treated with acute high-dose or chronic narcotics
2. The nature and intensity of the pain is not explained by a current or previous GI diagnosis**
3. ***Two or more*** of the following:
   a. The pain worsens or incompletely resolves with continued or escalating dosages of narcotics
   b. There is marked worsening of pain when the narcotic dose wanes and improvement when narcotics are re-instituted (soar and crash)
   c. There is a progression of the frequency, duration, and intensity of pain episodes

* Pain must occur most days

** A patient may have a structural diagnosis (e.g., inflammatory bowel disease, chronic pancreatitis), but the character or activity of the disease process is not sufficient to explain the pain

## E. Gallbladder and Sphincter of Oddi Disorders

### E1. BILIARY PAIN

*Diagnostic criteria*

Pain located in the epigastrium and/or right upper quadrant and ***all*** of the following:

1. Builds up to a steady level and lasts 30 minutes or longer
2. Occurring at different intervals (not daily)
3. Severe enough to interrupt daily activities or lead to an emergency department visit
4. Not significantly (<20%) related to bowel movements
5. Not significantly (<20%) relieved by postural change **or** acid suppression

*Supportive criteria*

The pain may be associated with:

1. Nausea and vomiting
2. Radiation to the back and/or right infra subscapular region
3. Waking from sleep

### E1a. Functional Gallbladder Disorder

*Diagnostic criteria* *Must include **both** of the following:*

1. Criteria for biliary pain*
2. Absence of gallstones or other structural pathology

*Supportive criteria*

1. Low ejection fraction on gallbladder scintigraphy
2. Normal liver enzymes, conjugated bilirubin, and amylase/lipase

* ***Criteria for biliary pain:*** Pain located in the epigastrium and/or right upper quadrant and **all** of the following: 1. Builds up to a steady level and lasts 30 minutes or longer. 2. Occurring at different intervals (not daily). 3. Severe enough to interrupt daily activities or lead to an emergency department visit. 4. Not significantly (<20%) related to bowel movements. 5. Not significantly (<20%) relieved by postural change **or** acid suppression.

### E1b. Functional Biliary Sphincter of Oddi Disorder

*Diagnostic criteria* *Must include **all** of the following:*

1. Criteria for biliary pain*
2. Elevated liver enzymes or dilated bile duct, but not both
3. Absence of bile duct stones or other structural abnormalities

*Supportive criteria*

1. Normal amylase/lipase
2. Abnormal Sphincter of Oddi manometry
3. Abnormal hepatobiliary scintigraphy

* ***Criteria for biliary pain:*** Pain located in the epigastrium and/or right upper quadrant and **all** of the following: 1. Builds up to a steady level and lasts 30 minutes or longer. 2. Occurring at different intervals (not daily). 3. Severe enough to interrupt daily activities or lead to an emergency department visit. 4. Not significantly (<20%) related to bowel movements. 5. Not significantly (<20%) relieved by postural change **or** acid suppression.

### E2. Functional Pancreatic Sphincter of Oddi Disorder

*Diagnostic criteria* *Must include **all** of the following:*

1. Documented recurrent episodes of pancreatitis (typical pain with amylase or lipase >3 times normal and/or imaging evidence of acute pancreatitis)
2. Other etiologies of pancreatitis excluded
3. Negative endoscopic ultrasound
4. Abnormal sphincter manometry

## F. Anorectal Disorders

### F1. Fecal Incontinence

*Diagnostic criterion**

Recurrent uncontrolled passage of fecal material in an individual with a developmental age of at least 4 years

* Criterion fulfilled for the last 3 months. For research studies, consider onset of symptoms of at least 6 months previously with two to four episodes of FI over 4 weeks

## F2. FUNCTIONAL ANORECTAL PAIN

### F2a. Levator Ani Syndrome

*Diagnostic criteria** *Must include **all** of the following:*

1. Chronic or recurrent rectal pain or aching
2. Episodes last 30 minutes or longer
3. Tenderness during traction on the puborectalis
4. Exclusion of other causes of rectal pain such as inflammatory bowel disease, intramuscular abscess, anal fissure, thrombosed hemorrhoids, prostatitis, coccygodynia, and major structural alterations of the pelvic floor

* Criteria fulfilled for the last 3 months with symptom onset at least 6 months prior to diagnosis

### F2b. Unspecified Functional Anorectal Pain

*Diagnostic criteria**

Symptom criteria for chronic Levator Ani Syndrome but no tenderness during posterior traction on the puborectalis muscle

* Criteria fulfilled for the last 3 months with symptom onset at least 6 months prior to diagnosis

### F2c. Proctalgia Fugax

*Diagnostic criteria** *Must include **all** of the following:*

1. Recurrent episodes of pain localized to the rectum and unrelated to defecation
2. Episodes last from seconds to minutes with a maximum duration of 30 minutes
3. There is no anorectal pain between episodes
4. Exclusion of other causes of rectal pain such as inflammatory bowel disease, intramuscular abscess, anal fissure, thrombosed hemorrhoids, prostatitis, coccygodynia, and major structural alterations of the pelvic floor

* For research purposes, criteria must be fulfilled for 3 months with symptom onset at least 6 months prior to diagnosis

## F3. FUNCTIONAL DEFECATION DISORDERS

*Diagnostic criteria** *Must include **all** of the following:*

1. The patient must satisfy diagnostic criteria for functional constipation and/or irritable bowel syndrome with constipation
2. During repeated attempts to defecate, there must be features of impaired evacuation, as demonstrated by ***two of the following three*** tests:
   a. Abnormal balloon expulsion test
   b. Abnormal anorectal evacuation pattern with manometry or anal surface EMG
   c. Impaired rectal evacuation by imaging

* Criteria fulfilled for the last 3 months with symptom onset at least 6 months prior to diagnosis

*Subcategories F3a and F3b apply to patients who satisfy criteria for FDD*

### F3a. Inadequate Defecatory Propulsion

*Diagnostic criterion**

Inadequate propulsive forces as measured with manometry with or without inappropriate contraction of the anal sphincter and/or pelvic floor muscles**

* Criterion fulfilled for the last 3 months with symptom onset at least 6 months prior to diagnosis

** This criterion is defined by age- and gender-appropriate normal values for the technique

### F3b. Dyssynergic Defecation

*Diagnostic criterion**

Inappropriate contraction of the pelvic floor as measured with anal surface EMG or manometry with adequate propulsive forces during attempted defecation**

* Criterion fulfilled for the last 3 months with symptom onset at least 6 months prior to diagnosis

** This criterion is defined by age- and gender-appropriate normal values for the technique

## G. Childhood Functional GI Disorders: Neonate/Toddler

### G1. Infant Regurgitation

*Diagnostic criteria* *Must include **both** of the following in otherwise healthy infants 3 weeks to 12 months of age:*

1. Regurgitation two or more times per day for 3 or more weeks
2. No retching, hematemesis, aspiration, apnea, failure to thrive, feeding or swallowing difficulties, or abnormal posturing

### G2. Rumination Syndrome

*Diagnostic criteria* *Must include **all** of the following for at least 2 months:*

1. Repetitive contractions of the abdominal muscles, diaphragm, and tongue
2. Effortless regurgitation of gastric contents, which are either expelled from the mouth or rechewed and reswallowed
3. ***Three or more*** of the following:
   a. Onset between 3 and 8 months
   b. Does not respond to management for GERD and regurgitation
   c. Unaccompanied by signs of distress
   d. Does not occur during sleep and when the infant is interacting with individuals in the environment

### G3. Cyclic Vomiting Syndrome (CVS)

*Diagnostic criteria* *Must include **all** of the following:*

1. Two or more periods of unremitting paroxysmal vomiting with or without retching, lasting hours to days within a 6-month period
2. Episodes are stereotypical in each patient
3. Episodes are separated by weeks to months with return to baseline health between episodes of vomiting

### G4. Infant Colic

*Diagnostic criteria For clinical purposes, must include **all** of the following:*

1. An infant who is less than 5 months of age when the symptoms start and stop
2. Recurrent and prolonged periods of infant crying, fussing, or irritability reported by caregivers that occur without obvious cause and cannot be prevented or resolved by caregivers
3. No evidence of infant failure to thrive, fever, or illness

"Fussing" refers to intermittent distressed vocalization and has been defined as "[behavior] that is not quite crying but not awake and content either." Infants often fluctuate between crying and fussing, so that the two symptoms are difficult to distinguish in practice.

*For clinical research, a diagnosis of infant colic must meet the preceding diagnostic criteria **and also include both** of the following:*

1. Caregiver reports infant has cried or fussed for 3 or more hours/day during 3 or more days in 7 days in a telephone or face-to-face screening interview with a researcher or clinician
2. Total 24-hour crying plus fussing in the selected group of infants is confirmed to be 3 hours or more when measured by at least one prospectively kept 24-hour behavior diary

### G5. Functional Diarrhea

*Diagnostic criteria Must include **all** of the following:*

1. Daily painless, recurrent passage of four or more large, unformed stools
2. Symptoms last more than 4 weeks
3. Onset between 6 and 60 months of age
4. No failure-to-thrive if caloric intake is adequate

### G6. Infant Dyschezia

*Diagnostic criteria Must include **both** of the following in an infant less than 9 months of age:*

1. At least 10 minutes of straining and crying before successful or unsuccessful passage of soft stools
2. No other health problems

### G7. Functional Constipation (FC)

*Diagnostic criteria Must include **one month of at least two** of the following in infants up to 4 years of age:*

1. Two or fewer defecations per week
2. History of excessive stool retention
3. History of painful or hard bowel movements
4. History of large diameter stools
5. Presence of a large fecal mass in the rectum

**In toilet-trained children, the following additional criteria may be used:**

6. At least one episode/week of incontinence after the acquisition of toileting skills
7. History of large diameter stools which may obstruct the toilet

## H. Childhood Functional GI Disorders: Child/Adolescent

### H1. FUNCTIONAL NAUSEA AND VOMITING DISORDERS

### H1a. Cyclic Vomiting Syndrome (CVS)

*Diagnostic criteria* *Must include **all** of the following:*

1. Two or more periods of intense, unremitting nausea and paroxysmal vomiting, lasting hours to days within a 6-month period
2. Episodes are stereotypical in each patient
3. Episodes are separated by weeks to months with return to baseline health between episodes
4. After appropriate evaluation, the symptoms cannot be attributed to another medical condition

### H1b. Functional Nausea and Functional Vomiting

#### *H1b1. Functional Nausea*

*Diagnostic criteria** *Must include **all** of the following:*

1. Bothersome nausea as the predominant symptom, occurring at least twice per week, and generally not related to meals
2. Not consistently associated with vomiting
3. After appropriate evaluation, the nausea cannot be fully explained by another medical condition

* Criteria fulfilled for at least 2 months prior to diagnosis

#### *H1b2. Functional Vomiting*

*Diagnostic criteria** *Must include **all** of the following:*

1. On average, one or more episodes of vomiting per week
2. Absence of self-induced vomiting or criteria for an eating disorder or rumination
3. After appropriate evaluation, the vomiting cannot be fully explained by another medical condition

* Criteria fulfilled for at least 2 months prior to diagnosis

### H1c. Rumination Syndrome

*Diagnostic criteria** *Must include **all** of the following:*

1. Repeated regurgitation and rechewing or expulsion of food that:
   a. Begins soon after ingestion of a meal
   b. Does not occur during sleep
2. Not preceded by retching
3. After appropriate evaluation, the symptoms cannot be fully explained by another medical condition. An eating disorder must be ruled out.

* Criteria fulfilled for at least 2 months prior to diagnosis

### H1d. Aerophagia

*Diagnostic criteria** *Must include* ***all*** *of the following:*

1. Excessive air swallowing
2. Abdominal distension due to intraluminal air that increases during the day
3. Repetitive belching and/or increased flatus
4. After appropriate evaluation, the symptoms cannot be fully explained by another medical condition

* Criteria fulfilled for at least 2 months prior to diagnosis

## H2. FUNCTIONAL ABDOMINAL PAIN DISORDERS

### H2a. Functional Dyspepsia (FD)

*Diagnostic criteria* *Must include* ***one or more*** *of the following bothersome symptoms at least 4 times a month for at least 2 months prior to diagnosis:*

1. Postprandial fullness
2. Early satiation
3. Epigastric pain or burning not associated with defecation
4. After appropriate evaluation, the symptoms cannot be fully explained by another medical condition

*Within FD the following subtypes are now adopted:*

***H2a1. Postprandial distress syndrome (PDS)*** includes bothersome postprandial fullness or early satiation that prevents finishing a regular meal. Supportive features include upper abdominal bloating, postprandial nausea, or excessive belching.

***H2a2. Epigastric pain syndrome (EPS)*** which includes all of the following: bothersome (severe enough to interfere with normal activities) pain or burning localized to the epigastrium. The pain is not generalized or localized to other abdominal or chest regions and is not relieved by defecation or passage of flatus. Supportive criteria can include (a) burning quality of the pain but without a retrosternal component, (b) commonly induced or relieved by ingestion of a meal but may occur while fasting.

### H2b. Irritable Bowel Syndrome (IBS)

*Diagnostic criteria** *Must include* ***all*** *of the following:*

1. Abdominal pain at least 4 days per month associated with ***one or more*** of the following:
    a. Related to defecation
    b. A change in frequency of stool
    c. A change in form (appearance) of stool
2. In children with abdominal pain and constipation, the pain does not resolve with resolution of the constipation (children in whom the pain resolves have functional constipation, not IBS)
3. After appropriate evaluation, the symptoms cannot be fully explained by another medical condition

* Criteria fulfilled for at least 2 months prior to diagnosis

### H2c. Abdominal Migraine

*Diagnostic criteria** *Must include **all** of the following occurring at least twice:*

1. Paroxysmal episodes of intense, acute periumbilical, midline or diffuse abdominal pain lasting 1 hour or more (should be the most severe and distressing symptom)
2. Episodes are separated by weeks to months
3. The pain is incapacitating and interferes with normal activities
4. Stereotypical pattern and symptoms in the individual patient
5. The pain is associated with ***two or more*** of the following:
   a. Anorexia
   b. Nausea
   c. Vomiting
   d. Headache
   e. Photophobia
   f. Pallor
6. After appropriate evaluation, the symptoms cannot be fully explained by another medical condition

* Criteria fulfilled for at least 6 months prior to diagnosis

### H2d. Functional Abdominal Pain – Not Otherwise Specified

*Diagnostic criteria** *Must be fulfilled at least 4 times per month and include **all** of the following:*

1. Episodic or continuous abdominal pain that does not occur solely during physiological events (e.g., eating, menses)
2. Insufficient criteria for irritable bowel syndrome, functional dyspepsia, or abdominal migraine
3. After appropriate evaluation, the abdominal pain cannot be fully explained by another medical condition

* Criteria fulfilled for at least 2 months prior to diagnosis

## H3. FUNCTIONAL DEFECATION DISORDERS

### H3a. Functional Constipation (FC)

*Diagnostic criteria* *Must include **two or more** of the following occurring at least once per week for a minimum of 1 month with insufficient criteria for a diagnosis of IBS:*

1. Two or fewer defecations in the toilet per week in a child of a developmental age of at least 4 years
2. At least one episode of fecal incontinence per week
3. History of retentive posturing or excessive volitional stool retention
4. History of painful or hard bowel movements
5. Presence of a large fecal mass in the rectum
6. History of large diameter stools, which can obstruct the toilet
7. After appropriate evaluation, the symptoms cannot be fully explained by another medical condition

**H3b. Nonretentive Fecal Incontinence**

*Diagnostic criteria* *Must include at least a 1-month history in a child with a developmental age older than 4 years of **all** of the following:*

1. Defecation in places inappropriate to the sociocultural context
2. No evidence of fecal retention
3. After appropriate evaluation, the fecal incontinence cannot be explained by another medical condition

## APPENDIX B

# Clinical Programs for DGBI

Listed below are medical programs that are committed to treat patients with DGBI. We selected these programs based on their credibility, resources, and the providers' scientific reputations. Each program is listed alphabetically by state in the USA and by country for international programs. We provide a brief description of each program, their website, the names of the providers, and the contact information for making an appointment.

## UNITED STATES

### North Carolina - *Durham*

### Drossman Gastroenterology

Drossman Gastroenterology specializes in helping patients with difficult to diagnose and treat DGBI and motility disorders, utilizing the biopsychosocial/patient-centered care model. The practice is led by Douglas A. Drossman (**https://theromefoundation.org/staff-member/douglas-a-drossman-md/**), who pioneered research, teaching the clinical practice of the DGBI. He founded and was past president of the Rome Foundation and was co-director of the UNC Center for Functional GI and Motility Disorders. His special interests include chronic abdominal pain, IBS, constipation, diarrhea, nausea and vomiting syndromes, pelvic floor disorders, and DGBI associated with severe psychosocial impact. He is recognized for the application of neuromodulators to manage symptoms that have not succeeded with traditional treatments.

***Website:*** **https://drossmancare.com/gastroenterology/**

***Making an Appointment:*** (919) 246-5611

***Our Provider:*** Douglas A. Drossman, MD

### Arizona - *Phoenix*

### Mayo Clinic - Scottsdale

The Motility Group and the Esophageal Group at Mayo Clinic Arizona are part of a nationally renowned Gastroenterology Group ranking #6 in the United States according to *US News & World Report* for 2020. We offer a full range of diagnostic and therapeutic services and are well-versed in disorders of gut-brain interaction as well as immune and nonimmune-mediated disorders of gastrointestinal function that may co-exist. In addition to managing GERD, dysphagia, noncardiac chest pain, dyspepsia, IBS, constipation, fecal incontinence, and pelvic floor dysfunction, we also work in a multidisciplinary approach to motility disturbances and their consequences such as SIBO and malnutrition.

We work in close collaboration with our surgical colleagues in cardiothoracic surgery, colorectal surgery, and urogynecology as well as with allied health, which includes dieticians with special training in GI disorders/low FODMAP/six-food elimination diet and physical therapists with special training in treating pelvic floor problems. Our therapeutic endoscopists are proficient at esophageal myotomy and G-POEM. We also work in close conjunction with our psychiatry department for help with neuromodulators and psychologists proficient with cognitive behavioral therapy to help manage the psychological impact of chronic disease.

***Website:*** **https://www.mayoclinic.org/departments-centers/gastroenterology-hepatology-digestive-care/home/orc-20348202**

***Making an Appointment:***
Lucinda Harris, MD
Phoenix, AZ – Mayo Clinic in Arizona
(800) 446-2279 (toll-free)
8 a.m. to 5 p.m. Mountain Standard Time, Monday through Friday
**https://www.mayoclinic.org/appointments**

**California – *Los Angeles***

**The Vatche and Tamar Manoukian Division of Digestive Diseases at UCLA**

A leader in disorders of gut-brain interaction (DGBI), we approach patient care through a paradigm in which the brain-gut axis is central to diagnosis and treatment. We view patients holistically—providing integrative care that combines the best pharmacological treatments with selected complementary therapies, including mind-body approaches. We offer a patient-centered program for patients suffering from DGBI. A multidisciplinary team that includes internationally renowned experts in brain-gut interactions works to better understand the causes, to pinpoint the problems, and to provide state-of-the-art care. Through a holistic approach to evaluation and treatment that involves doctors, nurses, and dietitians—built on a foundation of better understanding functional GI disorders through cutting-edge scientific studies and clinical trials leading to improved treatments—we are able to improve the lives of patients suffering from these conditions.

***Website:*** **https://www.uclahealth.org/gastro/ibs**

***Making an Appointment and Our Providers:***
Lin Chang, MD, or Kirsten Tillisch, MD
Westwood – GI, Suite 205 | (310) 208-5400
Lisa Lin, MD
Beverly Hills | (310) 855-7002
Lynn Connolly, MD
Santa Monica | (310) 582-6240

### Connecticut - *New Haven*

### Yale School of Medicine—Yale New Haven Health

The Functional Gastrointestinal Disorders Program at Yale New Haven Health is a new addition to its robust digestive health service line. Our team members have special training in disorders of gut-brain interaction, having worked with leaders in the field both nationally and internationally. We pride ourselves on an innovative and unique approach to complex patient care and work collaboratively with colleagues from nutrition services, behavioral health, and pelvic floor health including colorectal surgery, urogynecology, and physical therapy. Additionally, we work intimately with our colleagues in pediatric gastroenterology to transition adolescents with disorders of gut-brain interaction to adult gastroenterology providers.

***Website:*** **https://www.ynhh.org/services/digestive-health/functional-gastrointestinal-disorders.aspx**

***Making an Appointment (In Person or Telehealth):*** (203) 785-4138

***Our Provider:*** Jill Deutsch, MD

### Florida - *Jacksonville*

### Mayo Clinic - Jacksonville

Dr. Brian E. Lacy is a board-certified gastroenterologist who focuses his research and clinical interests on disorders of gastrointestinal motility. Dr. Lacy's areas of expertise include Gastroesophageal Reflux Disease (GERD), dysphagia, achalasia, dyspepsia, gastroparesis, Irritable Bowel Syndrome (IBS), constipation, intestinal pseudo-obstruction, and visceral pain.

***Website:*** **https://www.mayoclinic.org/**

***Making an Appointment:***
Mayo Clinic, Division of Gastroenterology
Davis Building, 6th Floor, 4500 San Pablo Road, Jacksonville, FL 32224
(904) 953-2594 | fax (904) 953-6225

***Our Provider:*** Brian E. Lacy, PhD, MD

### Illinois - *Chicago*

### Neurogastromotility and Interdisciplinary Bowel Dysfunction Programs at Northwestern University

The mission of the Northwestern Medicine Digestive Health Center (**nm.org/dhc**) is to prevent, diagnose, and treat disorders of the digestive tract and associated organs. At the heart of the Center's success is the complementary approach through multidisciplinary teams of providers who work to bring top-quality care to patients from around the world. Our center includes a sophisticated diagnostic motility laboratory and dedicated areas of specialization including the Esophageal program, the Interdisciplinary Bowel Dysfunction and Neurogastromotility programs (**https://nm.org/conditions-and-care-areas/gastroenterology/digestive-health-center/functional-bowel-disease-program**), and Behavioral Medicine. The NM DHC Behavioral Medicine program (**nm.org/gastrobmed**) in particular is one of the largest and most fully integrated Psychogastroenterology programs in academic medicine. Our providers, including licensed clinical psychologists and registered dieticians, work with DHC providers and patients to offer GI-focused Cognitive Behavioral Therapy, Gut-Directed Medical Hypnosis, brief solution focused therapies, Medical Nutrition Therapy, inpatient consultation, support groups, and training.

The Northwestern Medicine Digestive Health Center provides comprehensive care for a broad range of digestive health issues. Our patients benefit from the multidisciplinary programs which coordinate gastroenterologists, interventional endoscopists, surgeons, clinical psychologists, and registered dietitians, ensuring care for the whole patient and their families.

***Website:*** **https://nm.org/conditions-and-care-areas/gastroenterology/digestive-health-center/functional-bowel-disease-program**

***Providing Practitioners:*** **https://nm.org/conditions-and-care-areas/gastroenterology/digestive-health-center/functional-bowel-disease-program/meet-the-downtown-functional-bowel-neurogastromotility-team**

***Making an Appointment:*** (312) 695-5620

***Our Providers:***
John Pandolfino, MD (Gastroenterology)
Darren M. Brenner, MD (Gastroenterology)
Amy L. Halverson, MD (Colorectal Surgery)
Sarah E. Quinton, PsyD (Behavioral Medicine)
Kathryn N. Tomasino, PhD (Behavioral Medicine)
Sarah Kinsinger, PhD (Behavioral Medicine)
Anjali U. Pandit, PhD (Behavioral Medicine)
Bethany Doerfler, MS, RDN (Nutrition)
Amy Kassebaum, PA-C, RD, MMS (Gastroenterology APP)

## Indiana - *Carmel*

### Indiana University North Hospital GI Clinic

The clinic at IU North Hospital focuses on caring for patients with functional gastrointestinal and motility disorders such as Irritable Bowel Syndrome, Evacuation Disorders, Functional Constipation, and Gastroparesis. This clinic operates as part of a larger multi-disciplinary Motility Program at Indiana University led by Dr. John Wo with access to a fully equipped GI motility laboratory as well as two full-time GI psychologists who are trained in delivering highly specialized care to patients who suffer from disorders of the gut-brain axis. Our clinical program is integrated with an active neurogastroenterology and motility research program that focuses on novel diagnostic and therapeutic strategies care for patients who suffer from functional GI disorders, including those disorders that may be significantly affected by central dysregulation and psychological distress. We also have two PhD GI psychologists, Drs. Anne Mary Montero and Sean Jones.

***Website:*** **https://medicine.iu.edu/faculty/4791/shin-andrea**

***Making an Appointment:***

For Gastroenterology: 11725 N Illinois St, Suite 275; Carmel, IN 46032
(888) 484-3258

For GI Psychologist: IU Health Spring Mill Outpatient Center,
10300 North Illinois Street, Suite 1100
(317) 944-0980

***Our Provider:*** Andrea Shin, MD

## Maryland – *Baltimore*

### Johns Hopkins Motility Center

The Johns Hopkins Motility Center helps patients with difficult to diagnose and treat DGBI and motility disorders, utilizing the biopsychosocial/patient-centered care model. Dr. Stein has been providing clinical care at Hopkins for 10 years. The motility team works together to care for complex patients with a trained motility nurse practitioner, Valerie Owen, and a specialized nurse, Talia Jackowitz. Dr. Stein's special interests include pelvic floor and bowel control disorders including constipation and fecal incontinence as well as Irritable Bowel Syndrome. Dr. Stein also collaborates with ENT and head and neck radiation oncologists for complex care of oropharyngeal and esophageal swallowing disorders. Dr. Stein works closely with colleagues in physical therapy, urogynecology, surgery, nutrition, psychology, psychiatry, neurology, and rheumatology to provide comprehensive care.

***Website:*** **https://www.hopkinsmedicine.org/gastroenterology_hepatology/specialty_centers/motility_neurogastroenterology.html**

Motility and Neurogastroenterology | Johns Hopkins Division of Gastroenterology and Hepatology

***Making an Appointment:*** Please send records for review and then call to schedule: (410) 933-7495

***Our Providers:***

Ellen Stein, MD, Johns Hopkins Gastroenterology, Motility Team
Valerie Owen, NP, Johns Hopkins Gastroenterology, Motility Team
Talia Jackowitz, RN, Johns Hopkins Gastroenterology, Motility Team

## Massachusetts – *Boston*

### Beth Israel Hospital

Beth Israel Deaconess Medical Center utilizes a multi-disciplinary and collaborative approach to treating DGBI patients. Our team includes a GI psychologist and robust research program, as well as close collaborations with Women's Health and the Pelvic Floor Health Team. We conduct innovative research studies with new medications as well as non-drug alternative therapies.

***Website:*** **https://www.bidmc.org/centers-and-departments/digestive-disease-center/services-and-programs/ibs-and-functional-bowel-disorders-program/meet-our-team**

***Making an Appointment:*** (617) 667-8888

***Our Providers:***
Anthony Lembo, MD
Sarah K. Ballou, PhD, GI psychologist

## Michigan – *Ann Arbor*

### Michigan Medicine at University of Michigan

At Michigan Medicine, we have two programs for patients with DGBI and motility disorders. For patients with upper and lower digestive complaints like Functional Dyspepsia and Irritable Bowel Syndrome, we have the ***Functional Bowel Disorders Clinic***. The FBD group consists of highly trained gastroenterologists with an interest in DGBI and motility disorders. For patients with severe chronic constipation or fecal incontinence, we have the ***Michigan Bowel Control Program (MBCP)***. This program, founded in 2005, was one of the first in the US to take a multi-disciplinary, integrated approach to pelvic floor conditions. MBCP incorporates the expertise of specially trained gastroenterologists, uro-gynecologists, colorectal surgeons, and physical medicine, rehabilitation doctors, working shoulder-to-shoulder with specialized nurses, GI dietitians, gastropsychologists, and physical therapists to provide integrated, collaborative, multi-disciplinary care.

***Website:*** **https://www.uofmhealth.org/conditions-treatments/digestive-and-liver-health/make-gi-appointment**

***Making an Appointment:***
GI Clinic Call Center: (888) 229-7408
GI Behavioral Health Program: (888) 229-7408

***Our Providers:***
William D. Chey, MD, AGAF, FACG, FACP
Director, Digestive Disorders Nutrition & Behavioral Health Program
Megan E. Riehl, PsyD, GI Psychologist

## Minnesota - *Rochester*

### Mayo Clinic - Rochester

The Motility Group and the Esophageal Group at Mayo Clinic Rochester are part of a nationally renowned Gastroenterology Group ranking #6 in the United States according to *US News & World Report* for 2020. We offer a full range of diagnostic and therapeutic services and are well-versed in disorders of gut-brain interaction as well as immune and nonimmune-mediated disorders of gastrointestinal function that may co-exist. In addition to managing GERD, dysphagia, noncardiac chest pain, dyspepsia, IBS, constipation, fecal incontinence, and pelvic floor dysfunction, we also work in a multidisciplinary approach to motility disturbances and their consequences such as SIBO and malnutrition. We work in close collaboration with our surgical colleagues in cardiothoracic surgery, colorectal surgery, and urogynecology as well as with allied health, which includes dieticians with special training in GI disorders/low FODMAP/ six-food elimination diet and physical therapists with special training in treating pelvic floor problems. Our therapeutic endoscopists are proficient at esophageal myotomy and G-POEM. We also work in close conjunction with our psychiatry department for help with neuromodulators and psychologists proficient with cognitive behavioral therapy to help manage the psychological impact of chronic disease.

***Website:*** **https://www.mayoclinic.org/departments-centers/gastroenterology-hepatology-digestive-care/home/orc-20348202**

***Making an Appointment:***
Mayo Clinic Gastroenterology and Hepatology
200 First St. SW, Rochester, MN 55905
(507) 284-2511
**https://www.mayoclinic.org/appointments**

***Our Providers:***
Madhu Grover, MD
Jean Fox, MD

## Missouri - *St. Louis*

### Washington University School of Medicine in St. Louis Division of Gastroenterology

Our center has a specialty Neurogastroenterology and Motility section that provides advanced diagnostic modalities, including high manometric and advanced physiologic testing as well as comprehensive therapeutic options including biofeedback, pelvic floor therapy, cognitive behavioral, hypnotherapy, and acupuncture approaches as well as extensive experience with conventional and novel pharmacotherapies. Our Center is also recognized by the American Neurogastroenterology and Motility Society (ANMS) as a Clinical Training Program Center of Excellence.

***Website:*** https://gastro.wustl.edu

***Making an Appointment:*** Ms. Beth Buschard-Steiger, (314) 454-8201

***Our Providers:***
C. Prakash Gyawali, Professor of Medicine
Washington University School of Medicine / Barnes-Jewish Hospital
**https://gastro.wustl.edu/faculty/chandra-prakash-gyawali-md-mrcp/**
Dr. Gregory Sayuk, Associate Professor of Medicine and Psychiatry
Washington University School of Medicine / St. Louis VA Medical Center
**https://gastro.wustl.edu/faculty/gregory-s-sayuk-md-mph/**
Dr. Cheryl Richards, Associate Professor of Medicine and Psychiatry
Washington University School of Medicine / Barnes-Jewish Hospital
**https://gastro.wustl.edu/faculty/cheryl-richards-phd/**

## New York – *New York City (Manhattan)*

### Susan Lucak, MD

Dr. Susan Lucak's approach to patient care is to listen carefully to patients' symptoms and concerns. She performs a targeted work-up without excessive testing. During office visits a considerable amount of time is spent on educating patients about their conditions and on encouraging them to be involved in their own care. Dr. Lucak believes that patient-physician relationship requires a teamwork approach and over the years this has resulted in the best outcomes.

Dr. Lucak has focused her practice on disorders of gut-brain interaction, including Irritable Bowel Syndrome, Chronic Abdominal Pain, persistent diarrhea, chronic constipation, and bloating among others. She involves dieticians, psychologists, pelvic floor physical therapists, and psychiatrists in the care of her patients as appropriate.

***Website:*** www.lucakmd.com

***Making an Appointment:***
903 Park Avenue, First Floor, New York, NY 10075
(212) 861-0481

***Our Provider:*** Susan Lucak, MD

## North Carolina – *Chapel Hill*

### University of North Carolina Gastroenterology Program

We provide expert consultations and ongoing care for patients with a full spectrum of acute and chronic gastrointestinal conditions, from the simple to the complex. Over 17,000 visits are made annually, with 100–150 new patient visits each month. Among those treated in our clinic, 95% are very satisfied and 96% would recommend us to a friend. Ongoing programs aim to continuously improve quality of care and patient experience across clinical programs. Anne Peery is one of the faculty with particular interest in treating patients with disorders of gut-brain interaction.

***Website:*** **https://www.med.unc.edu/medicine/gi/patient-care/clinical-services/general-gastroenterology-clinic/**

***Making an Appointment:***
(984) 974-5050 | fax (984) 974-3414

***Our Provider:*** Anne Peery, MD

## North Carolina – *Charlotte*

### Atrium Health Motility Clinics

Our specialists at Atrium Health Motility Clinics help with management of patients with chronic gastrointestinal diseases and have a wide range of expertise. Our team manages Functional Dyspepsia, Gastroparesis, constipation, IBS, and many rare and common disorders whether functional or due to a motility disorder. We also offer diagnostic testing and management by a GI psychologist where necessary, which helps our patients by providing a comprehensive and multidisciplinary approach to chronic and unaddressed issues.

***Website:*** **https://atriumhealth.org/medical-services/specialty-care/other-specialty-care-services/atrium-health-gastroenterology-and-hepatology**

***Making an Appointment:***
1025 Morehead Medical Drive, Suite 300, Charlotte, NC
(704) 355-4593 | fax (704) 355-2485

***Our Providers:***
Baharak Moshiree, MD, MS-c
  Director of Motility at Atrium Health
  Morehead Medical Plaza
Mackenzie Jarvis, MPAM, DMSc, PA-C
  Instructor in the Department of Internal Medicine
  Atrium Health Gastroenterology and Hepatology
Jason Baker, PhD
  Physiology and Motility Lab Technical Director
  Assistant Professor Atrium Health, Department of Medicine and Department of Surgery
Elyse Thakur, PhD
  GI psychologist
  Faculty in Atrium Health

## North Carolina – *Winston-Salem*

### GI Neuromuscular Disorders Program at Wake Forest Baptist Medical Center

The GI Neuromuscular Disorders Program at Wake Forest Baptist Medical Center is directed by Nyree Thorne, MD. Consultation services with Dr. Thorne, Steven Clayton, MD, and Kenneth Koch are available and a full range of motility testing is offered.

***Making an Appointment:***
To schedule consultations or tests, (336) 713-7777

***Our Providers:***
Esophageal Motility Disorders: Steven Clayton, MD
Gastric Motility Disorders: Kenneth Koch, MD
Colon and Colorectal Motility Disorders: Nyree Thorne, MD

## Ohio – *Cleveland*

### The Esophageal and Swallowing Center (ESC) and the Neurogastroenterology and Motility Program (NMP), MetroHealth System

The ESC and NMP specialize in providing patients with DGBI state-of-the-art and cutting-edge testing and a comprehensive therapeutic approach that includes medical, behavioral, nutritional as well as alternative and complementary medicine. The ESC is led by Ronnie Fass, MD, who dedicated his long career to the understanding of DGBI of the upper gut. The NMP is led by Gengqing Song, MD, PhD, who has general interest in DGBI and specifically in acupressure and transcutaneous electrical acupoint stimulation.

***Website:*** **https://www.metrohealth.org/gastroenterology**

***Clinic address:*** Main Campus, 2500 MetroHealth Drive, Cleveland, OH 44109
Parma, 12301 Snow Road, Parma, OH 44130

***Making an Appointment:*** (216) 778-5736

***Our Providers:***
Ronnie Fass, MD
Gengqing Song, MD, PhD
Tanja Barco, APRN-CNP
Buddy Ross

## Texas – *Houston*

### The Ertan Digestive Disease Center at Memorial Hermann-Texas Medical Center and The University of Texas Health Science Center at Houston (McGovern Medical at UTHealth) Medical School

This center provides comprehensive medical and surgical treatment for patients with diseases of the esophagus, stomach, intestine, pancreas, biliary tract, and liver. Offering access to the leading treatment options available, patients have the full support of a top-ranked comprehensive hospital in the world-renowned Texas Medical Center. Under the care of affiliated physicians, patients receive innovative and effective multidisciplinary gastroenterology treatments. The goal is to provide excellence in clinical care and research, delivering outstanding patient care with compassion and a strong background of cutting-edge clinical research in gastroenterology and hepatology. They provide expert management, up-to-date treatment and innovative solutions for patients with all forms of digestive disorders, and continually work to enhance patient quality of care as well as improve quality of life for their patient population.

***Website:*** **http://www.memorialhermann.org/locations/texas-medical-center/ertan-digestive-disease-center/**

***Making an Appointment:***
Ertan Digestive Disease Center-Texas Medical Center
6400 Fannin Street, #1400, Houston, TX 77030
(800) 985-4837 | (713) 704-3450 | fax (713) 704-9938

***Our Provider:*** Brooks Cash, MD

## Texas – *Houston*

## Houston Methodist

Our team of physicians, nurses, and other healthcare professionals work together to diagnose and treat digestive disorders, including diseases of the esophagus, stomach, liver, pancreas, biliary (gallbladder, bile ducts, and bile) tree, small intestine, and colon, with leading-edge technology and research. Houston Methodist's advanced treatment options, psychological support, pain management, rehabilitation, and palliative care all add up to a comprehensive approach and personalized experience that begins with your very first visit. Houston Methodist physicians collaborate in the fields of gastroenterology, surgery, oncology, and radiology to ensure that patients receive comprehensive, innovative, and compassionate care. Our gastroenterologists and gastrointestinal surgeons use sophisticated, state-of-the-art imaging technologies to evaluate the physiology of the gastrointestinal (GI) tract, assisting in diagnosis and the latest and most comprehensive treatment options.

***Website:*** **https://www.houstonmethodist.org/gastroenterology/services/**

***Making an Appointment:***
Smith Tower, 6550 Fannin St. Ste 1201, Houston, TX 77030
(713) 441-3372
**https://www.houstonmethodist.org/request-an-appointment/patient/?physician=eamonn-quigley&pcg=false**

***Our Provider:*** Eamonn Quigley, MD

## UNITED STATES – PEDIATRIC GASTROENTEROLOGY

**Connecticut – *Hartford***

**Connecticut Children's Medical Center**

We offer pediatric gastroenterology research-based care (**https://www.connecticutchildrens.org/search-specialties/gastroenterology/**) to children, teenagers, and young adults with a broad range of digestive system disorders. Connecticut Children's is among the most active in the country for basic, clinical, and translational research (**https://www.connecticutchildrens.org/search-specialties/gastroenterology/gastroenterology-research/**). Our Center for Neurogastroenterology and Motility Disorders (**https://www.connecticutchildrens.org/search-specialties/gastroenterology/gastroenterology-programs-services/center-for-neurogastroenterology-and-motility-disorders/**) offers specialized interventions, clinics, and therapies for a large variety of disorders of gut-brain interaction.

***Website:*** www.connecticutchildrens.org

***Making an Appointment:*** (860) 545-9560

***Our Provider:*** Jeffrey Hyams, MD

**Florida – *Miami***

**University of Miami/Comprehensive Motility & Abdominal Pain Center**

At the Comprehensive Motility & Abdominal Pain Center at the University of Miami/Holtz Children's Hospital, we are dedicated to improving the lives of our patients and families through personalized diagnostic and treatment options. Our team uses a multidisciplinary approach, which includes nutritionists, psychologists, social workers, child life specialists, and complementary medicine when appropriate. Our center is led by Dr. Miguel Saps, world-renowned pediatric motility specialist and Co-Chair of the Pediatric Rome Committee and includes three experts in pediatric neurogastroenterology.

***Website:*** https://pediatrics.jacksonhealth.org/services/pediatric-gastroenterology-hepatology-nutrition/

***Making an Appointment:***
(305) 243-3166 or email PediatricGI@med.miami.edu

***Our Provider:*** Miguel Saps, MD

**Massachusetts – *Boston***

**Boston Children's Hospital**

**Center for Motility and Functional Gastrointestinal Disorders**

The Center not only provides state-of-the-art care and evaluation for children with motility and functional bowel disorders, but has a well-funded research base, as well as a well-defined educational component that allows the training of the next generation of pediatric gastrointestinal (GI) motility specialists. Dr. Nurko has distinguished himself during his long tenure as an academic, NIH-funded clinical researcher, teacher, mentor, and expert in motility and functional disorders of the gastrointestinal tract in children. Dr. Nurko has made major contributions to the understanding of motility and functional GI disorders in children. His clinical and research interests have focused on understanding the pathophysiology and establishing the best approach and treatments for these disorders, and he has been a pioneer in the development and validation of new techniques to study these disorders in the pediatric population.

***Website:*** **http://www.childrenshospital.org/**

***Making an Appointment:***
Center for Motility and Functional Gastrointestinal Disorders
Boston Children's Hospital
300 Longwood Ave., Boston, MA 02115
(617) 355-6055

***Our Provider:*** Samuel Nurko, MD

**North Carolina - *Chapel Hill***

**UNC Children's, Division of Pediatric Gastroenterology, DGBI Program**

The UNC Children's DGBI Program provides interdisciplinary care using the biopsychosocial model for pediatric patients under 18 years of age with Disorders of Gut-Brain Interaction (DGBI), including diagnosis and treatment of conditions such as Functional Abdominal Pain, Functional Dyspepsia, Irritable Bowel Syndrome, Functional Nausea and Vomiting, and Cyclic Vomiting Syndrome. Treatment recommendations may include use of neuromodulator and other medications, psychological therapies, and nutrition support services. Program psychologists provide diagnostic and consultative services, brief intervention, and referral for evidence-based therapies for DGBI.

***Website:*** **www.uncchildrens.org/uncmc/unc-childrens/care-treatment/gastroenterology-hepatology**

***Making an Appointment:*** (919) 966-2435

***Our Providers:***
Rose C. Marcus, MD, MSCE, Pediatric Gastroenterologist
Camden E. Matherne, PhD, Pediatric Psychologist
Joni McKeeman, PhD, Pediatric Psychologist
Lisa Richardson, MS, RD, Pediatric Dietitian

**Ohio - *Columbus***

**Nationwide Children's Hospital, Center for Neurogastroenterology and Motility Disorders**

The Center for Neurogastroenterology and Motility Disorders at Nationwide Children's Hospital is well established and recognized as one of the world's premier centers for the care of children with DGBI and motility disorders. The practice is multidisciplinary and involves six pediatric gastroenterologists, dedicated psychologists, nurse practitioners, a physician assistant, and nurses who are all trained to care for children and adolescents with DGBI and motility disorders. The center is led by the medical director Desale Yacob, MD, and its director Carlo Di Lorenzo, MD. There is a dedicated multidisciplinary DGBI clinic that provides comprehensive care to children with Chronic Abdominal Pain, IBS, Functional Dyspepsia, nausea, and other DGBI. The long-standing and successful rumination therapy program is the only one of its kind in the country. The center is also one of the first to start a neuromodulation program with gastric electric and sacral nerve stimulation. The center has programs for biofeedback therapy and bowel management including one for children with autism. The motility providers are active members of the Center for Colorectal and Pelvic Reconstruction (CCPR), a center that excels in providing multidisciplinary and comprehensive surgical care to children with anorectal malformations. A referral from the patient's medical provider is required for an appointment.

***Website:*** **https://www.nationwidechildrens.org/specialties/motility-center**

***Clinic Address:*** GI Division, Motility Center
700 Children's Drive, Columbus, OH 43205

***Making an Appointment:*** (614) 722-3456

***Our Providers:***
Carlo Di Lorenzo, MD, Director
Desale Yacob, MD, Medical Director
Neetu Bali, MD, MPH
Peter Lu, MD, MS
Karla Vaz, MD, MEd
Kent Williams, MD
Ashley Kroon Van Diest, PhD
Kim Osborne, DNP
Anita Fouch, DNP
Jody Wall, PA-C

### Texas – *Houston*

### Texas Children's Hospital

The Multidisciplinary Abdominal Pain Program (MAPP) Clinic at Texas Children's Hospital provides patient-centered consultation services for children with abdominal pain due to disorders of gut-brain interaction. Created out of a partnership between the Anesthesia Pain Medicine and Neurogastroenterology programs at Texas Children's, the MAPP Clinic uses an integrated team consisting of a pain medicine specialist, pain psychologist, and gastroenterologist with support from dietitians and physical therapists to provide care consistent with the biopsychosocial model.

***Websites:***

https://www.texaschildrens.org/departments/pain-medicine

https://www.texaschildrens.org/departments/neurogastroenterology-and-motility-program

https://www.bcm.edu/research/labs-and-centers/research-centers/childrens-nutrition-research-center/research/labs/pediatric-abdominal-pain

***Email:*** Dr. Andrew Chu, andrew.chu@bcm.edu

***Making an Appointment:*** (832) 824-7246 [PAIN]

***Our Provider:*** Dr. Andrew Chu

## INTERNATIONAL

### Australia – *Sydney*

### John Hunter Hospital

Dr. Nick Talley, MD, PhD, is a senior staff specialist gastroenterologist at the John Hunter Hospital-Royal Newcastle Centre and Distinguished Laureate Professor at the University of Newcastle. He staffs a dedicated weekly outpatient clinic and endoscopy list. This service provides care to patients with digestive disorders with a focus on unexplained GI diseases including functional dyspepsia, IBS and IBD, constipation, and esophageal disorders. This service is supported by a GI Fellow and dietician.

***Email:*** HNELHD-ReferralCentre@hnehealth.nsw.gov.au

***Making an Appointment:***
Outpatient Service – North Block, Level 2, John Hunter Hospital
Lookout Rd, New Lambton Heights, NSW 2305
phone: (02) 4922 3912

***Our Provider:*** Nicholas Talley, MD, PhD

### Beijing – *China*

### Clinic for FGID/DGBI, Peking Union Medical College Hospital (PUMCH)

Our hospital is the earliest and the most influential center to provide integrative care for FGID/DGBI patients in China. The FGID team consists of four professors and one associate professor from Department of Gastroenterology, one associate professor from Department of Geriatrics, and one associate professor from Department of Psychological Medicine. The GI motility center can provide a comprehensive evaluation for GI function and biofeedback therapy. We apply a convenient two-way referral between gastroenterologist and psychologist, follow-up appointment, and a multidisciplinary consultation for difficult patients. Patients may select a consulting physician in different clinic places like regular clinic, special need clinic, and international medical clinic.

***Making an appointment for international medical clinic:***
***Website:*** **https://www.pumch.cn/en/medical_care.html**
***Hotline:*** phone: 86-10-69156699

***Making an appointment for regular clinic and special need clinic:***
Please download PUMCH APP

***Our Providers:***
Meiyun Ke, MD
Xiucai Fang, MD
Liming Zhu, MD
Guijun Fei, MD
Xiaoqing Li, MD
Xiohong Sun (Geriatrics), MD
Lili Shi (Psychological Medicine), MD

## Belgium – *Leuven*

## Leuven University Hospital Division of Gastroenterology/Hepatology – Neurogastroenterology and Motility Clinic

The Neurogastroenterology and Motility Clinic at Leuven University Hospital is a multidisciplinary outpatient clinic that focuses on the management of patients with difficult to diagnose and treat DGBI and motility disorders. Patients are evaluated by experienced gastroenterologists with an interest in these disorders, and have access to all state-of-the-art diagnostic and supportive measures. The clinic was founded by Prof. Jan Tack, who has published extensively on these conditions, and who is president of the Rome Foundation. Additional leading clinicians in the Neurogastroenterology and Motility Clinic at Leuven University Hospital are Prof. Tim Vanuytsel, Prof. Guy Boeckxstaens, Prof. Philip Caenepeel, Prof. Joris Arts, and Dr. Frederik De Clerck.

***Website:*** **https://www.uzleuven.be/en**

***Making an Appointment:*** phone: (+32) (0)16344225

***Our Providers:***
Prof. Jan Tack
Prof. Tim Vanuytsel
Prof. Guy Boeckxstaens
Prof. Philip Caenepeel
Prof. Joris Arts
Dr. Frederik De Clerck

## Brazil – *Porto Alegre*

## Carlos Francisconi, MD

Carlos Francisconi is a physician dedicated to caring for patients with functional gastrointestinal disorders including chronic abdominal pain, IBS, constipation, diarrhea, dyspepsia, nausea and vomiting syndromes, and DGBI associated with severe psychosocial impact. He has great experience in the field and has participated in multiple regional, national, and international meetings as lecturer on these topics.

***Making an Appointment:***
R. Ramiro Barcelos 910/902
Porto Alegre, Rio Grande do Sul, Brazil
phone: (51) 32221344

***Our Provider:*** Carlos Francisconi, MD

**Canada – *Ontario, Toronto***

**University Health Network (UHN) Motility Clinic**

The UHN Motility Clinic specializes in the diagnosis and management of various disorders of gut-brain interaction (such as irritable bowel syndrome, functional dyspepsia, etc.) and motility disorders. The clinic offers advanced motility testing including esophageal manometry, ambulatory pH monitoring, and anorectal manometry. The clinical team includes physicians, a nurse clinical care coordinator, and a dietitian who specializes in gastrointestinal disorders. In addition to providing clinical care, our program conducts clinical research in the field of disorders of gut-brain interaction and is involved in educating the next generation of clinicians to care for patients with these conditions.

***Website:*** https://www.uhn.ca/MCC/Clinics/Motility_Clinic

***Making an Appointment:***
Referrals must be sent from a physician to fax: 416-603-5039
399 Bathurst St. 4th floor East Wing, Toronto, Ontario, M5T 2S8

***Our Providers:***
Louis W.C. Liu, MD, PhD, FRCPC
Yvonne Tse, MD, FRCPC
Colleen Parker, MD, FRCPC

**Chile – *Santiago***

**CEDIF (Digestive Center for Functional GI Disorders)**

CEDIF is a center specializing in treating patients with difficult to diagnose DGBI and motility disorders. We use the biopsychosocial/patient-centered care model of care. The practice is led by Freddy Squella Boerr, MD, and includes a GI psychologist and physical therapy professionals. Our special interests include chronic abdominal pain, IBS, constipation, diarrhea, nausea and vomiting syndromes, pelvic floor disorders, and DGBI associated with severe psychosocial impact.

***Website:*** www.cedif.cl

***Making an Appointment:*** phone: 22-343-1158

***Our Provider:*** Freddy Squella Boerr, MD

## India - *Lucknow*

### Luminal Gastroenterology, Functional GI diseases, and GI Motility Services, Department of Gastroenterology, Sanjay Gandhi Postgraduate Institute of Medical Sciences

For Luminal Gastroenterology including functional GI disease educational services for the patients and doctors, Prof. Ghoshal uses **www.biomedinfo.net** and **www.spreadhealth.in**. Group Awareness for Patients (GAP) sessions are held regularly for patient education.

***Making an Appointment:*** phone: Mr. Prashant Singh, +91-9455773837 or +91-8004590796

***Our Provider:*** Dr. Uday Ghoshal

## Iran - *Isfahan*

### FNM Clinic, Al-Zahra Hospital of Isfahan University

This is a collaborative interdisciplinary GI-Psyche OPD service that is located in Salamat Building, Al-Zahra Hospital of Isfahan University of medical sciences. Each patient may be consulted in a meeting by a group of specialists. Mostly referral/refractory cases are accepted. The setting is academic and covers educational and research activities as well. In case of essence the patient may also benefit from in-patient psychosomatic ward care.

***Making an Appointment:*** phone: 00983136202093

***Our Providers:***

Dr. Peyman Adibi, GI Clinic

Diagnosis and treatment; primary encounter and medical care by a specialist as well as easy access to consultations by Dr. Hassan Shahoon, a GP who is practically and academically trained for psychosomatic care in functional disorders. There is also optional dietary consultation by Dr. Mohammadi (Phd in nutrition) when needed.
32°37'37.7"N 51°39'51.6"E

Dr. Hamid Afshar/Dr. Elham Shirzadi Psychiatry Clinic

They provide psychiatric consult and design pharmacotherapy for GI-referred cases and follow-up of psychiatric disorders along with symptomatic treatment of DGBI, and plan further investigation and interventions regarding basic and advanced psychchosomatic care including inpatient care.
32°37'34.1"N 51°39'53.1"E

Parsian Psychology Center by Dr. Moghtadaie

Psychological therapies are tailored for each individual based on his/her background symptom/disorder including stress management training, CBT, ACT, and family therapy.
32°37'44.5"N 51°39'59.7"E

## Israel – *Tel Aviv*

### Gastromed Specialist Clinics

Our clinic provides diagnosis and treatment for DGBI patients, with hypnotherapist, CBT psychologists, nutritionist, and pelvic floor therapists available.

***Website:***
Hebrew: **https://www.gastromed.co.il/גסטרומד-אונליין/**
English: **https://www.gastromed.co.il/english/gastromed-english/welcome-to-gastromed/**

***Making an Appointment:***
Weizman 14, Tel Aviv, 14th floor, Rm 1401
phone: 03-6970700 or from abroad +97236970700

***Our Provider:*** Ami Sperber, MD, MSPH
**https://www.pro-digestion.com**

## Italy – *Bologna*

### University of Bologna (NGM-UNIBO)

The Neurogastroenterology and Motility Center at the University of Bologna (NGM-UNIBO), based at S. Orsola Hopital in Bologna, Italy, builds on a long-lasting tradition of excellence in gastroenterology. Our clinical activities and patient care are strongly intertwined with research and teaching. NGM-UNIBO is one of the busiest referral centers for FGID in Italy and certified by the Italian National Institute of Health as the referral center for rare forms severe dysmotility syndromes (e.g., chronic intestinal pseudo-obstruction). At NGM-UNIBO, a team of experts performs specialist visits for inpatients and outpatients and assessment of gastrointestinal motility, sensitivity, microbiota, epithelial permeability, food intolerances, and allergies with state-of-the art equipment, including high resolution manometry, breath tests, and an in-house patented test for the diagnosis of gluten sensitivity. Patients can take advantage of therapeutic approaches including traditional, novel, and experimental therapies, including also biologics and intestinal microbiota transplantation.

***Making an Appointment:*** phone: +39.051 214 4916 or +39.051 214 4100

***Our Providers:***
Professor Vincenzo Stanghellini, (email) **v.stanghellini@unibo.it**
**https://www.unibo.it/sitoweb/v.stanghellini/cv-en**
Professor Giovanni Barbara, (email) **giovanni.barbara@unibo.it**
**https://www.unibo.it/sitoweb/giovanni.barbara/en**

## Italy – *Milan*

### Clinical Institute Humanitas

The University-led Operating Unit deals with the prevention, diagnosis, and medical and/or endoscopic treatment of digestive diseases (esophagus, stomach, small intestine, colon, anorectum, pancreas, and biliary tract).

***Website:*** **https://www.humanitas.it/unita-operative/gastroenterologia**

***Making an Appointment:*** phone: +39 02 82241

***Our Provider:*** Enrico Stefano Corazziari, MD, **www.enricocorazziari.it**

***Email:***
For information in English submit requests to **enrico.corazziari@uniroma1.it**
Pour information en Francais ècrivez a **enrico.corazziari@uniroma1.it**

**Italy** – ***Rome***

**Studio Medico Villa Massimo**
**Casa di Cura Pio XI**

Both Centers offer biopsychosocial, environmental-centered care for patients with chronic gastrointestinal, neurogastroenterological, and inflammatory conditions. Highly-qualified dietary counselling, endoscopic-histologic, and functional gastrointestinal (pH-impedentiometry-manometry) investigations are available. Online gastroenterological and dietary counselling are also available.

***Website:***
**http://www.casadicurapioxi.it/medici?764caa40-cafa-4ee6-ab0e-1e712e2781f6**

***Making an Appointment:***
Studio Medico Villa Massimo, phone: +39 06 44243298
Casa di Cura Pio XI, phone: +39 06 664941

***Our Provider:*** Enrico Stefano Corazziari, **www.enricocorazziari.it**

**Italy** – ***Verona***

**GI Physiology and Motility Disorders Unit of the University of Verona, AOUI Verona**

The Unit is devoted to evaluation and management of patients with functional gastrointestinal disorders unresponsive to standard care. The upper GI physiology is tested by high resolution manometry and PH24HrsImpedenziometry. Lower GI is studied by high resolution manometry, Pelvic Floor EMG, and balloon expulsion test. Food intolerances are acknowledged by lactose and fructose breath test as well as small bowel bacterial overgrowth and delayed transit by glucose and lactulose breath test. Rome Criteria are extensively used on diagnosis to favor cooperative management of the difficult patient. Management of swallowing and defecation disorders is enhanced by dedicated biofeedback techniques developed onsite. Pelvic pain is also considered among disorders suitable of behavior techniques. Gut-oriented hypnotherapy is reserved for selected IBS and functional dyspepsia groups of patients where alternative management has failed.

***Email:*** **chiarioni@hotmail.com**

***Making an Appointment:*** phone: Ms. Sandra Rizzi, Lab Tech, +390458126405

***Our Providers:***
Giuseppe Chiarioni, MD, RFF
Francesca Cidoni, RN
Sandra Rizzi, Lab Tech

**Japan – *Sendai***

**Department of Psychosomatic Medicine, Tohoku University Hospital**

We are a representative center for the care of Irritable Bowel Syndrome (IBS) in Japan. Patients are treated with a biopsychosocial approach.

***Website:*** **http://www.hosp.tohoku.ac.jp/sinryou/s08_sinryou.html**

***Making an Appointment:*** phone: Ms. Moriyama, +81-22-717-7734

***Our Providers:***
Shin Fukudo, MD, PhD
Motoyori Kanazawa, MD, PhD. Email **m-kanazawa@med.tohoku.ac.jp**

**Malaysia – *Universiti Sains Malaysia, Kota Bharu***

**My Gut-Brain Center**

We are based in Malaysia with a clinical program encompassing consultancy, products, research, education, and training. Focus areas include neuro-gastroenterology (GI Function and Motility Unit, Hospital USM), functional GI disorders, gut microbiota, and solutions to gut-brain disorders. The team is led by Professor Yeong Yeh, Justin LEE, MD, PhD.

***Website:*** **www.mygutbraincenter.com**

***Making an Appointment:*** **gifunctionmotility@gmail.com**

***Our Provider:*** Professor Yeong Yeh, Justin LEE, MD, PhD

**Mexico – *Mexico City***

**Located at Clinica Lomas Altas, S.C.**

Dr. Max Schmulson, MD, is a gastroenterologist who specializes in Functional Gastrointestinal Disorders and Motility of the Gastrointestinal Tract. Clinical consultations and manometry studies are available.

***Making an Appointment:***
Avenida Paseo de la Reforma #2608
Piso 9. Col. Lomas Altas, C.P. 11950
**gastrolomas@yahoo.com.mx**
phone: 52-5562859600; 52-5562859603

***Our Provider:*** Max Schmulson, MD

**Romania – *Cluj-Napoca***

**Badeamedica**

Clinic for ambulatory gastroenterological patients including endoscopy, ultrasonography, and psychosomatic counselling/CBT psychotherapy.

***Website:*** **http://badeamedica.ro/medici/**

***Making an Appointment:***
Manager: Ana Damian, Str. Rene Descartes Cluj-Napoca, 400486 Romania
Email: **office@badeamedica.ro**
phone +40 364 140 260; +40 757 530 367

***Our Provider:*** Prof Dan L. Dumitrascu, MD, PhD

**Romania – *Cluj-Napoca***

**Clinica Medicala 2, Cluj-Napoca, Romania (2nd Medical Dept., Cluj County Clinical Hospital, Iuliu Hatieganu University of Medicine and Pharmacy Cluj-Napoca, Romania)**

This is a tertiary center specializing in internal medicine and gastroenterology, with special focus on DGBI and GI motility disorders. Patients are seen in ambulatory, day hospitalization, or continuous hospitalization. Psychogastroenterological management is also offered. Considered the most experienced center for DBGI in Romania and very influential in Central and East Europe. Complete gastroenterological workup and laboratory for functional gastrointestinal investigations.

***Website:*** **https://scjucluj.ro/index.php/sectii-si-compartimente/sectii-compartimente/61-medicina-interna-iii**

***Making an Appointment:***
Prof. Dan L. Dumitrascu: **ddumitrascu@umfcluj.ro**, phone/fax: + 40264593355
Liliana David, PhD, RN: **lilidavid2007@yahoo.com**, secretariat

***Our Provider:*** Prof. Dan L. Dumitrascu, MD, PhD

**Singapore**

**Stomach, Liver & Bowel Clinic**

The Stomach, Liver & Bowel Clinic at Gleneagles Hospital is led by Kok-Ann Gwee, MBBS, FAMS (Gastroenterology), FRCP, PhD. He is a leading authority on irritable bowel syndrome (IBS) and constipation. In addition to the management of stomach, liver, and bowel disorders, Dr. Gwee provides expertise in the management of Dyspepsia, indigestion, gas-related complaints, bowel habit training and dietary management of food intolerance, refractory GERD and *H. pylori* infection, and small intestinal bacterial overgrowth. His specific hepatology interests are the management of fatty liver and Hepatitis E.

***Website:*** www.drgwee.com

***Making an Appointment:***
Gleneagles Hospital Annexe Block
6A Napier Road Suite #05-37, Singapore 258500
phone: (65) 6474 6848 | fax: (65) 6475 8285 | answering service: (65) 6535 8833
Email: **admin@drgwee.com**

***Our Provider:*** Dr. Kok Ann Gwee, MBBS (Singapore), M Med (Internal Medicine), MRCP (UK), PhD (Sheffield), FAMS (Gastroenterology), FRCP (London), FRCP (Glasgow)

**Sweden** – ***Gothenborg***

**Neurogastroenterology Unit**

The Neurogastroenterology Unit (Swedish name: "Mag – och tarmlaboratorium") is a specialized unit for diagnostic tests, treatment, and clinical research for patients with functional gastrointestinal disorders (FGID) or disorders of gut-brain interaction (DGBI). A wide range of therapeutic and educational resources can be offered at the unit. Professor Magnus Simrén and Associate Professor Hans Törnblom are together with Gisela Ringström, RN, PhD, co-chairing the unit. There are also several specialized nurses, physicians, and dietitians working at the unit. Several clinical research projects, including different treatment trials, run simultaneously at the unit.

***Website:*** **https://www.sahlgrenska.se/omraden/omrade-6/specialistmedicin/enheter/mag-och-tarmlaboratorium/**

***Email:*** magtarmlab.su@vgregion.se

***Making an Appointment:*** phone: 031-342 81 07

***Our Providers:***
Magnus Simren, MD, PhD
Hans Törnblom, MD

**United Kingdom** – ***London***

**The Neurogastroenterology Group**

The Neurogastroenterology Group is a multidisciplinary collaboration of experts, both clinicians and scientists, including adult and paediatric neurogastroenterologists, physiologists, psychologists and psychiatrists, and surgeons, working across the Blizard Institute, Barts and The London School of Medicine and Dentistry, and Barts Health NHS Trust to enhance patient care through research and innovation. We have clinical and research expertise in visceral pain, GI Neuromuscular disorders, Gastroesophageal Reflux Disease, colorectal disease, nausea and appetite, surgical innovation, drug discovery, and other novel areas. Each programme is led by a theme leader.

***Website:*** **https://www.qmul.ac.uk/blizard/research/research-groups/neurogastroenterology-group/#d.en.420528**

***Making an Appointment:***
Barts and the London School of Medicine and Dentistry
Queen Mary University of London
4 Newark St, London, E1 2AT
**qmul.ac.uk/blizard/**
phone: +44(0)20 7882

***Our Providers:***
Prof. Qasim Aziz, Phd, FRCP
Prof. Charles H. Knowles, BChir, PhD, FRCP

**United Kingdom –** ***Nottingham***

**Nottingham Neurogastroenterology Unit**

The Nottingham Neurogastroenterology Unit is led by Dr. Maura Corsetti and consists of a Clinic, where gastroenterologists with training and interest in Functional Gastrointestinal Disorders evaluate and treat patients, and a Motility Lab, where high-resolution esophageal manometry, 24hr pH-impedance, anorectal manometry, balloon expulsion test, transanal ultrasound, antroduodenal manometry, colonic manometry, Oddi's sphincter manometry, electronic barostat, and breath tests are performed. The Unit is linked with a Medical Physics Lab, where scintigraphic gastric emptying, and small bowel and colonic transit evaluation are performed; with a dedicated outpatient dietician service; with a Behavioral and Rehabilitation unit, where a multidisciplinary team of behavioral psychologists/psychiatrists and physical therapists coordinate rehabilitation and rectal irrigation outpatient clinic; and with a Pelvic unit where gastroenterologists, gynecologists, urologists, neurologists, radiologists, and colorectal surgeons collaborate for the evaluation and treatment of patients with pelvic disorders.

***Making an Appointment:*** Send an email to **maura.corsetti@nuh.nhs**

***Website:*** **https://nddcbru.org.uk/**

***Our Provider:*** Dr. Maura Corsetti

**Uruguay –** ***Montevideo***

**Clínica de Gastroenterología, Universidad de la República**

Clínica de Gastroenterología is a department of the public university medical school that aims to assist, teach, and research in Gastroenterology, Hepatology, and GI endoscopy. It is a national reference center and in its external consultation more than 3500 patients are assisted annually, many of them with functional disorders. Its Neurogastro lab includes lactose and lactulose breath tests, manometry, and impedance-pH monitoring. Using a multidimensional approach and a multidisciplinary team (gastroenterologists, nutritionists, psychologists, and psychiatrists), patients with functional disorders are treated and followed up.

***Program Director:*** Carolina Olano, MD, MSc (Edu), AGAF

***Website:*** **http://www.gastro.hc.edu.uy/gastro/**

***Email:*** clinicagastrouru@hc.edu.uy

***Making an Appointment:***
Hospital de Clínicas
Av. Italia s/n. CP 11600, Montevideo, Uruguay
phone: +598 24808472

***Our Provider:*** Carolina Olano, MD, MSc (Edu), AGAF

## PSYCHOLOGICAL SERVICES

### GastroPsychology

**The Rome GastroPsych group** was founded in 2017 with the goal of connecting clinicians and scientists from around the world interested in brain-gut psychotherapies and the psychosocial aspects of DGBI. Ample evidence from large, randomized controlled trials supports the use of brain-gut psychotherapies for a wide range of DGBI. These therapies have been adapted from existing effective psychological treatments to focus specifically on gastrointestinal symptoms and their psychological sequelae. Common brain-gut psychotherapies are GI-focused cognitive behavior therapy (GI-CBT) and gut-directed hypnotherapy. **Membership** in the group is limited to professionals, who can gain access to our professional listserv, basic and advanced training programs, treatment manuals, research mentorship and collaboration and networking opportunities. To date the group has >300 members, and includes mental health providers, physicians, and advanced practice providers.

***Website:*** For a searchable list of providers, visit Rome Foundation GastroPsych **https://romegipsych.org**

## APPENDIX C

# Educational Products and Resources

## DIGITAL PRODUCTS

**GI Genius:** The GI Genius Interactive Clinical Decision Toolkit is a cloud-based program that provides an online resource to assist in the diagnosis and treatment of DGBI for adults and children. It combines the Rome IV Diagnostic Algorithms and the Rome IV Multidimensional Clinical Profile (MDCP). It also includes a full component of diagnostic and treatment algorithms of pediatric patients and an improved psychosocial navigation section, including content on the use of neuromodulators.

**Communication 101** is an innovative video learning tool developed by DrossmanCare for doctors who work with patients having DGBI. It is also valuable for patients who want to understand in just a few minutes of information about their medical disorders. This program leverages the expertise of 15 experts in neurogastroenterology to demonstrate how they educate patients with DGBI on the most common clinical issues that arise in the course of a clinical visit. Included in this program are 32 educational discussions, covering 11 content categories. The interviews are brief, only 3–8 minutes, and include a detailed written statement describing what was said and why. For some topics, more than one clinician demonstrates their approach so the learner can select which method best fits their style.

**Communication 202:** This innovative video learning tool developed by DrossmanCare teaches the sophistication and complexity of the medical interview. The program demonstrates educational techniques to improve communication skills, patient-centered care, psychosocial assessment, shared decision making, and methods to optimize the patient-provider relationship. The medical symptoms are only the entry point to explore in greater depth the patient's understanding, associated psychological features, patient concerns and behaviors, and at a deeper level, the psychosocial derivatives of the illness that drives the clinical presentation.

The program consists of six clinical vignettes each with four components to guide in the learning:

1. An ineffective interview where the physician makes errors in communication leading to a negative clinical interaction. The visit does not provide meaningful clinical information and leads to mutual dissatisfaction of patient and doctor.
2. A patient-centered facilitative interview that discloses more meaningful information and leads to the discovery of important underlying clinical information and psychosocial factors. This leads to patient and doctor satisfaction.
3. An interview with the patient discussing his or her perceptions of the previous two interviews. The discussion includes what the patient liked and didn't like about the physician's style.

4. A detailed step-by-step analysis of the interview including the key verbal and nonverbal messages. The narrator reviews worked and didn't work with regards to engaging with the patient and establishing a productive patient-doctor relationship.

## BOOKS

***Gut Feelings: Disorders of Gut-Brain Interaction and the Patient-Doctor Relationship***
Douglas A. Drossman, MD, and Johannah Ruddy, MEd

This book, endorsed by the Rome Foundation, educates patients and providers on the science, diagnosis, and treatment of DGBI and offers guidelines for patients and doctors to optimize the patient-doctor relationship. There are four sections:

Part 1. A Conceptual Understanding of the History, Philosophy, and Scientific Basis for the Disorders of Gut-Brain Interaction (DGBI)
Part 2. The Disorders of Gut-Brain Interaction (DGBI)
Part 3. Maximizing the Patient-Doctor Relationship
Part 4. What the Doctor Is Doing, or Should Be Doing

Published by DrossmanCare 2021.

**Rome IV, Volumes 1 & 2:**
***Rome IV Functional Gastrointestinal Disorders: Disorders of Gut-Brain Interaction (Fourth Edition)***
Douglas A. Drossman, MD, Lin Chang, MD, William D. Chey, MD, John Kellow, MD, Jan Tack, MD, PhD, and William Whitehead, PhD

The Rome IV textbook is a comprehensive update of knowledge in DGBI within a 1,500-page, two-volume book created by 117 internationally recognized clinicians and investigators in the field. Volume I contains background chapters on neurogastroenterology (basic science and physiology); pharmacology, pharmacokinetics, and pharmacogenomics; age, gender, women's health, and the patient's perspective; cross-cultural aspects of DGBI; the role of the micro-environment (food and microbiota); and biopsychosocial aspects of assessment and management. Volume II provides the key clinical information on 33 adult and 17 pediatric DGBI from esophagus to anorectum. For each DGBI we provide information on the epidemiology, pathophysiology, and psychosocial aspects as well as recommendations on diagnosis and treatment. Volume II discusses all the adult and pediatric DGBI. Published by the Rome Foundation 2016.

***Rome IV Diagnostic Algorithms for Common GI Symptoms (Second Edition)***
Douglas A. Drossman, MD, Lin Chang, MD, William D. Chey, MD, John Kellow, MD, Jan Tack, MD, PhD, and William Whitehead, PhD

This book focuses on how to make a diagnosis of all DGBI. There are eight chapters that help the reader understand the pathophysiology of the symptoms based on the area of symptoms and then moves on to diagnostic algorithms. Each algorithm includes features that bring the information to clinical reality: a) a case report linked to the algorithm in order to demonstrate real-life application, b) a color-coded graphic using standard "yes-no" decision tree methodology for branched decision making, c) links for each box to information that explains in detail the reasons for the clinical decision or the diagnostic assessment method and d) up-to-date references to support the clinical information. Published by the Rome Foundation 2016.

***Rome IV Multidimensional Clinical Profile (MDCP) for Functional Gastrointestinal Disorders (Second Edition)***
Douglas A. Drossman, MD, Lin Chang, MD, William D. Chey, MD, John Kellow, MD, Jan Tack, MD, PhD, and William Whitehead, PhD

This book teaches how doctors should treat patients with DGBI. It features over 70 clinical disorders and then guides the doctor to understand the complexity and dimensionality of these disorders. Just making a diagnosis is not sufficient to determine treatment. For example, a patient with mild and occasional symptoms of abdominal discomfort and loose stools and functioning without impairment would be treated quite differently than a patient with the same diagnosis having continuous severe and disabling pain and psychological distress with fears of incontinence when leaving the house. Published by the Rome Foundation 2016.

***Rome IV Functional Pediatric Functional Gastrointestinal Disorders: Disorders of Gut-Brain Interaction***
*Guest editors:* Carlo di Lorenzo, MD, and Sam Nurko, MD
*Editors:* Douglas A. Drossman, MD, Lin Chang, MD, William D. Chey, MD, John Kellow, MD, Jan Tack, MD, PhD, and William Whitehead, PhD

This book has an introduction by two well-known pediatric gastroenterologists who served as co–guest editors: Samuel Nurko, MD, from Harvard Medical School and Carlo Di Lorenzo, MD, from Ohio State University. The book contains updated and expanded pediatric chapters of the Rome IV book, a series of pediatric Multidimensional Clinical Profile (MDCP) cases for the Rome IV book, and a set of diagnostic algorithms for both neonate-toddlers and children-adolescents. This is a complete but compact book on DGBI for doctors seeing pediatric patients with DGBI. Published by the Rome Foundation 2016.

***Rome IV Functional Gastrointestinal Disorders for Primary Care and Non-GI Clinicians***
*Guest editors:* Joel Hedielbaugh, MD, and Pali Hungin, MD
*Editors:* Douglas A. Drossman, MD, Lin Chang, MD, William D. Chey, MD, John Kellow, MD, Jan Tack, MD, PhD, and William Whitehead, PhD

This book contains the Rome IV information about DGBI that is written for primary care doctors. The 12 chapters cover the spectrum of DGBI, but in a fashion that addresses the diagnoses most commonly seen, with emphasis on "how to" diagnosis and treatment information. Chapters first address the burden of DGBI on the patient and their relation to other functional somatic syndromes. Following this are the diagnostic and management strategies for primary care, patient-centered approaches to care, and then an understanding of these disorders from a biopsychosocial perspective. The second part addresses the most important DGBI: esophageal, gastroduodenal (functional dyspepsia), bowel (e.g., IBS and constipation), anorectal (e.g., dyssynergic defecation and incontinence), childhood disorders for neonates-toddlers and children-adolescents, centrally mediated disorders of GI pain (e.g., chronic pain and narcotic bowel syndrome), and finally multicultural aspects of DGBI. Published by the Rome Foundation 2016.

## EDUCATIONAL RESOURCES

**DrossmanCare – Chapel Hill, NC, USA**

DrossmanCare consists of an educational program (**www.drossmancenter.com**) to teach doctors and patients biopsychosocial, patient-centered care and communication skills, a specialty Neurogastroenterology practice (**www.drossmangastroenterology.com**), and a program for investors who want to enhance the reach of the educational mission (**www.drossmancare.com/investor-information**). DrossmanCare accepts healthcare providers who wish to visit the practice for mentoring and coaching as part of the Visiting Scholar Program (**https://drossmancare.com/gastroenterology/for-physicians/mentoring-coaching/**). The website provides written materials, blogs, videos, and other learning tools.

For information about educational programs and activities or to make contributions contact Johannah Ruddy (**jruddy@theromefoundation.org**).

**Rome Foundation / DrossmanCare Communication Skills Program**

Learn more about the Rome Foundation and DrossmanCare collaboration to produce educational resources, and guides to improve the patient-doctor relationship. Go to our website at **https://theromefoundation.org/programs-projects/rome-foundation-communication-program/** to find helpful downloads, videos, and other resources to assist both patients and doctors to better communicate in and outside of the clinical visit.

**GI Health Psychology**

Learn more about our Rome Foundation GastroPsych section by visiting our website at **https://theromefoundation.org/rome-gi-psych-committee/**. There you will find more about the role of health psychology in treating patients with DGBI, our GI Psychology Provider Directory, and other helpful resources for clinicians and patients.

**Rome University**

Learn more about our continuing education programs for clinicians treating patients with DGBI—both in-person and online. Our programs offer engaging and up-to-date learning opportunities with the world's leading experts in the field. See more on our website at **https://theromefoundation.org/cme**.

**International Foundation for Gastrointestinal Disorders (IFFGD)**

IFFGD is a registered nonprofit education and research organization. Our mission is to inform, assist, and support people affected by gastrointestinal (GI) disorders. IFFGD was founded in 1991 by one person struggling with the challenges imposed by a chronic GI disorder. Many others, from all walks of life, have joined with us. We work with patients, families, physicians, nurses, practitioners, investigators, regulators, employers, and others to broaden understanding about GI disorders, support or encourage research, and improve digestive health in adults and children. IFFGD has a wealth of resources on chronic gastrointestinal disorders including eight websites (iffgd.org, AboutIBS.org, AboutGERD.org, AboutGastroparesis.org, AboutConstipation .org, AboutGIMotility.org, AboutIncontinence.org, and AboutKidsGI.org), over 300 free downloadable fact sheets, and are active on all social media platforms. You can contact at **iffgd@iffgd.org**.

**Gastro Girl, Inc.**

Gastro Girl, Inc., empowers patients to achieve optimal digestive health. Gastro Girl offers resources such as evidence-based health information, access to an online patient education community via ginondemand.com, webinars, podcasts and more. Visit **https://gastrogirl.com**.

**GI OnDEMAND**

We are a gastroenterology virtual care and support platform. A joint venture between Gastro Girl and The American College of Gastroenterology, GI OnDEMAND provides healthcare providers and patients access to vetted GI expert registered dietitians, GI psychologists, and genetic counselors. Patients also have access to evidence-based health information and support resources including an online patient education community. Visit **https://giondemand .com/**.

**IBS Patient Support Group**

A dependable community to inform and support Irritable Bowel Syndrome (IBS) sufferers since 1987. Complete with evidenced-based medical causes, symptoms, support and treatment for digestive health sufferers, family and friends. Includes a community forum to share symptoms, treatment for constipation and diarrhea and diet, including the low FODMAP diet. Also incorporates the latest news related to IBS and personal patient diaries. Visit **www.ibspatient.org**.

**Tuesday Night IBS**

Tuesday Night IBS is a patient and clinician platform on both Twitter and Facebook that provides the opportunity for patients and clinicians to learn from each other. Each Tuesday night at 7pm ET, a guest host will tweet about a topic related to IBS—diet, new drug therapies, the role of gastropsychologists, the burden of illness, and more. We present case studies, the latest research data that is relevant to IBS for patients to know about, and offer a safe space for patients to share their own experiences and ask questions. Our Facebook page expands on that and provides videos, articles, and other resources.
Find us @TuesdayNightIBS on Twitter and Facebook.

**Douglas Drossman @DDrossman**
**Johannah Ruddy @JohannahRuddy**

Dr. Drossman and Ms. Ruddy follow the trends in DGBI research and clinical care providing information for patients and doctors. Follow them on Twitter and Facebook: @DDrossman and @JohannahRuddy

## INTERNATIONAL EDUCATIONAL RESOURCES

**Italy**

The nonprofit association "Associazione per la NeUroGastroenterologia e la Motilità Gastrointestinale" (ANEMGI-Onlus) mission is to promote research, education, and assistance for visceral dysfunctions caused by nervous system alterations and psychological and environmental conditions. Find more at **anemgi.org**.

**Japan**

Japanese Society of Gastroenterology (JSGE) is an academic organization that belongs to the Japanese Medical Association. JSGE provides comprehensive IBS guidelines for clinicians and patients. Find Clinical Practice Guidelines for Patients with Irritable Bowel Syndrome by Japanese Society of Gastroenterology at **https://www.jsge.or.jp/guideline/**.

## United Kingdom

The IBS Network is the UK's national charity supporting people with irritable bowel syndrome. We understand how difficult and embarrassing it can be to talk about symptoms. We know how symptoms can impact on your life and how miserable they can make you feel. You are not alone. We offer you support, advice, and information to help you live a full and active life again.

Visit our website **www.theibsnetwork.org** for more information to help you better self-manage your IBS. Alternatively, call 0114 272 3253.

# Index

Page numbers in *italics* refer to figures and tables.

Printed in Great Britain
by Amazon

81723969R00133